D0925377

THINK YOUNG!
FEEL YOUNG!
BE YOUNG!

The health secrets of the amazing Hunzas will bestow vitality, energy, and well-being. No matter your age or physical condition, the Hunza way to youth and health will give definite improvements in amazingly short time. Eat the Hunza way. Exercise the Hunza way. Live the Hunza way—the way to incredible physical and mental well-being.

The
Hunza-Yoga Way
to Health & Longer Life

Only by understanding the wisdom of the
body shall we attain that mastery of disease
and pain which shall enable us to relieve the
burden of mankind.

William Harvey, M.D.

THE HUNZA-YOGA WAY TO HEALTH AND LONGER LIFE

RENÉE TAYLOR

LANCER BOOKS ♞ NEW YORK

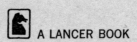 A LANCER BOOK

THE HUNZA-YOGA WAY TO HEALTH AND LONGER LIFE

This Lancer edition is published by arrangement with
Constellation International. Its large sale in the
high-priced hardcover edition makes possible this
inexpensive reprint.

To the Royal Family of Hunza
and its people, who have shown
me the way of life and truth

LANCER BOOKS, INC. • 1560 BROADWAY
NEW YORK, NEW YORK 10036

Contents

ACKNOWLEDGMENTS

I wish to express my appreciation and gratitude to all those who stood by me while I was writing this book, for their loyalty and interest in my work.

To Alice Cobb, who took all the pictures for this book, donating her time and effort to this project, as she felt yoga has done so much for her.

To Tom Abbott, Marsha Carr, Ann Dunn, Phyllis Samson, and Josette Guerne, who assist me in teaching yoga in Southern California, and whose pictures demonstrating the exercises appear throughout the book.

To Jessie Agena, Jean Ball, Roxy Reed, and Chris Dunn (twelve years old), my faithful students, for doing the various exercises.

I dedicate this book to the people of the world, as a gift of freedom and peace, as the yoga way of thinking has opened the door to a healthier and more confident living for me and so many of my students. Yoga has changed our lives to a better existence.

Renee Taylor

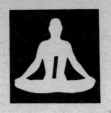

Introduction

WHY I BECAME INTERESTED IN YOGA

I remember it was a quiet afternoon. I was all alone in my lovely home in Hollywood, swimming in the pool. The shadows of the sun played joyfully on the flower beds and the green lawns.

Peace had descended on the place. I gave a sigh of relief and whispered aloud, "What fun, an afternoon to myself!" Usually this house is buzzing with people. People in and out. A pool in your back yard is an added attraction, and many wanderers come in for a dip. Few are concerned—even whether they are welcome.

I floated in the pool and sank into an oblivion, dreaming of yesterday. Suddenly the doorbell broke the silence. "Who could it be?" I was annoyed.

Still in my bathing suit, dripping, I opened the front door. A young man—neat and good-looking—stood there with a friendly smile on his face. "I'd like to demonstrate a soup to you. This is a very tasty and a very nourishing soup!" he said.

"I don't like soup! And besides young man, I am alone in the house and wouldn't let you in." I was determined.

"I don't want your home—just your kitchen facilities." This was even more absurd.

"No," I answered firmly.

But he was firm, too. "Please let me in. My story might interest you."

I could have banged the door in front of him, but something inside of me stopped me from doing it.

The door ajar, the stranger followed me to the kitchen. And in a few minutes he had the situation well in hand. A pot of water was boiling, two cups were on the table with some funny green-looking stuff in them. Then he poured the water over the powder and the soup was ready.

I must admit it tasted heavenly. The second cup followed. I praised his soup and my new friend became a little more at ease.

"You don't look well," he said to me. "Such a beautiful home and I wonder whether you are enjoying it."

He was right. It had been almost a year now that my health had been steadily going down. The doctor under whose treatment I had been for quite a while couldn't determine what was wrong. My blood pressure was very low, I was anemic, had constant trouble and pain during menstrual periods, headaches, dizzy spells. . . . A feeling of tiredness was all over my body and my ambition was down to zero. Getting out of bed in the morning became a real torture. I was also constantly short of breath. A few different injections three times a week seemed to help temporarily, but the next day I was depressed and tired again. Finally the doctor suggested an operation. I was not convinced I needed it and was thus undecided.

The stranger interrupted my thoughts. "The soup has food value. It is a concentrated vegetable powder. It supplies the body with additional strength and energy. Health food stores have it!"

"Health food stores. What are they? Drug stores? I've never heard about them or visited one."

"No, these are stores where you can buy all kinds of food—all natural foods, essential to your well-being."

Never before had I shopped in one of these so-called health food stores—and I asked many questions of him. I was curious to find out about them.

But then he was gone, leaving the soup on the table. "I haven't even paid you," I called out after him, but he was nowhere in sight. The jar on the table reminded me he was real. Otherwise, I would have thought it was a dream.

The next day I visited a health food store. What fun it was to read the labels! I discovered so many new things. I was always convinced I knew so much about my health and my body, but let me confess that I suddenly realized how ignorant I had been for such a long time. It was a great shock to me.

We are not aware of our bodies until something happens to them. Until then we abuse our health in the most ridiculous way. I learned so much during that first trip to the health food store. We would never dare to feed our animals with the foods prepared for our family. Our pets get special care, special foods, scientifically prepared according to formulas. We feed animals at a certain time, and give them nothing in between. The question comes up . . . Why do we take such good care of our animals and not of our children or ourselves?

Suddenly I realized that health begins in the kitchen. From there I began to build my own empire. I had so much to learn it was almost frightening. All my cupboards were cleaned out of the food I used to eat, replaced with natural whole grain cereals, brown rice, honey, and all kind of seeds, such as pumpkin seeds, sunflower seeds, sesame seeds, and natural oils, whole wheat flour, and so on.

The refrigerator, too, was filled with fresh vegetables, fresh juices, and many other tasty foods. People have such a wrong idea about health foods. They make fun of something they have never tasted. Just try once a deliciously prepared meal the health way, and you'll know the difference.

One Thanksgiving Day I invited a number of people for dinner. They confessed after the meal that they had been quite worried about getting some grass and had almost stopped to eat on the way. Needless to say, they were pleasantly surprised to get a delicious turkey with many other goodies. But everything was prepared the natural way.

With confidence I started rebuilding my own health. My faith began to mount. I knew that what I was doing was right. You have to have faith, otherwise you are defeated before you even begin. Even my thinking was changing. Naturally, I was far from being well, but I was feeling better.

So many of us walk through life half asleep, while life could be so bountiful and so magnificent. My "angel" who had started me on the road to good health has not reappeared . . . and I wonder whether he will ever learn how grateful I'll always be to him for putting some common sense into my stale brain.

HOW I WAS INTRODUCED TO YOGA!

It began one day when a dear friend of mine connected with the motion picture industry, the late Alice Field, asked me to have lunch with her. On our way to the restaurant we stopped to see Indra Devi, a yoga teacher. As we entered the room there were a few ladies doing some peculiar postures on the floor, and the petite teacher standing in front of the group was explaining the meaning of each twist and stretch, and what these exercises are supposed to be good for.

"Yoga, a simple method of physical fitness, will help you to overcome nervous tension, give you peace of mind, a better posture, control your weight problem . . . in other words, improve health and contribute to a longer life." It sounded too simple to be possible. I was skeptical, and to accept something that sounded so easy and so simple was quite difficult. And a skeptic is usually negative—and I was negative. So I shrugged my shoulders and this was that. . . .

Days went by and I forgot the episode. But destiny had another plan in store for me. One evening Indra Devi walked into my life again. She gave me a yoga lesson. When I saw her demonstrating the various postures with ease and comfort, I wanted to do the same, especially the lotus pose. But she said "No! Not yet. It takes a long time to accomplish this particular pose. It took me many months when I studied in India to sit this way." I was disappointed, but had no desire to argue. After all, she was the teacher.

That evening I gave much thought to everything she had told me. I was puzzled how these simple stretching and twisting postures can influence the working of the internal mechanism. Nevertheless, I had to admit that after the lesson I felt much more relaxed and at peace within myself.

That night I had an extraordinary dream. I was in India, at an *Ashram* (school), doing all the complicated exercises, including the lotus pose, the yoga-mudra, the headstand, and even the peacock. It was a wonderful experience and I woke up perfectly relaxed and happy, a feeling I hardly remembered for some time, due to my poor health. I knew something had happened that would lead me to find the way to health and peace.

And this is how yoga was introduced to me. It was obvious I was destined to study, and then to teach, to share it with others.

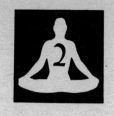

Hunza

Then I stumbled on the people of Hunza. It was during my visit to New York in 1952. I heard Dr. Maxwel O. Garten speak on nutrition, diets, and good health. In his talk he brought up the Hunza people as an example of the healthiest people on earth. Never before had I heard about them. They live, as I found out, high in the Himalayan Mountains and enjoy a long and happy life, without disease, to a ripe old age. Childhood diseases are virtually unknown. And these people also enjoy life without any crime and everyone obeys the law. They exist without a police force or jails, or army . . . so difficult to believe in our day of turmoil, riots, and crime.

But Dr. Garten's personality was so convincing he left no doubt in anybody's mind that it must be true. Even I began to melt. His ideas about health were revolutionary to my way of thinking. His road to good health led through water fasting. And his idea of eating was to keep the body healthy and nourished, not eating just for enjoyment.

"The Hunza people often have to fast at the end of the season when food runs out and there is nothing available but water," Dr. Garten told us. "But their water is pure, clean, coming from the mountains, full of minerals. Actually it is melted snow from the glaciers bringing all the rich minerals with it."

"If these people are so healthy, why can't it be done in our society?" I questioned Dr. Garten.

"Because people are skeptical. And besides it is so much more fun to complain about one's aches and pains," the doctor said with a smile.

"Oh, nonsense, I don't like to be ill," I said.

"Maybe you don't, but many people enjoy getting sympathy

from their husbands or family. People like to feel sorry for themselves."

On second thought I had to admit there was some truth in his words. I remembered that occasionally even I enjoyed playing the weak and ill female role. I am sure my husband watching me wondered whether it was for real.

"Do you think if anyone ate a simple diet and fasted once a year, the way the Hunza people do, it could improve his health or keep him healthy at all ages?" My thoughts were running fast.

"Of course!" He reassured me. "But people are lazy. Very few are interested in doing the right things. It takes time to lead a healthy life, and some planning, too. It is easier to be bad than good. And when it means work, so many shy away from it. But it can be done."

Although, I felt slightly better, I was far from being well. . . . "I'll fast, too! If these people are so healthy, why can't it be done in our society?" The thought ran through my mind. I still didn't tell the doctor about my aches and ill health. Ethics among the medical profession would demand that he get in touch with my doctor. This I wanted to avoid if possible.

And so I began to climb the new road to health. First I went on a twelve-day water fast, following his exact instructions. (In the chapter on fasting the details will be explained.) After that I planned my diet according to the Hunza way of eating. (You'll find the details in the chapter on diets and foods.)

Soon my taste for foods had radically changed. I began to enjoy meals prepared the natural way. More vegetables and fresh fruits, mostly raw, were included in my daily menus. Besides, I also started to take vitamins and minerals in tablet form. My health began steadily to improve and in a few months my pains were gone. My thoughts were so positive, there was no place for any negative thinking, or for complaints. Life took on a different meaning. There was a purpose to exist and look forward to a tomorrow. I was ready to build my new house on solid ground, leaving behind the past as forgotten history.

So far I haven't explained where Hunza is and who the people are who live there. Let me take you along with me on a journey to Hunza.

It is a mecca for all who seek good health along with a bonus of aesthetic beauty. You don't see medieval castles or cathedrals, but many spots have histories dating back to the time before Christ, and somehow the surrounding country looks as though it had been long lived in and loved. It has a kind of smile about it, an air of well-being, as unmistakable as it is pleasing.

For centuries, rumors of an earthly paradise high in the Himalayas have trickled through to the outside world, inspiring many great poets and authors to write of utopias—lands of ideal perfection. In our own time, James Hilton has written a book, *Lost Horizon*, about such a land which he called "Shangri-La," a make-believe spot where people enjoyed long and happy lives free from the complexities of modern times.

In the year 1961, I organized an expedition to join me on a trip to Hunza. We were six all together. My publishers called me "the modern Marco Polo" when they became aware of my ambitious venture.

The high Himalayas lift themselves in gleaming craggy symmetry and tower like snow-girdled symbols of the timeless valley that they surround and protect. Mount Rakoposhi, the Himalayan "Goddess of the Snows," lifts her ice-sheathed summit 25,550 feet into the darkening sky. This was Hunza Valley! This was Shangri-La! Jazz, neon lights, traffic, and all the teeming sounds that we Westerners naïvely label "civilization" were left behind.

There was a quietness in the mountain air. I became lost in this majestic slice of nature, where the flavor of tradition was so alive. Small terraced fields stretched upward from the valley floor like giant steps on the hillsides. Streets and canals were carefully cut around the terraced fields and trees. Those long, narrow canals scooped out by glaciers and the beautifully built garden terraces, symmetrically climbing up the mountain slopes, make a markedly civilized effect.

A few houses hidden by trees straggle up the slopes on either side; they stand proudly looking over the valley. All around them the gigantic mountains give a feeling of protection. And each spot has a charm of its own. What a superb site, an inspiring place for those who are privileged to live there.

But the beauty of this remote valley was not the reason for my being there. I was there to learn, to see, and experience. I felt I had to meet these people, otherwise my life wouldn't be complete. I used to say, "If I do nothing else in my life but go to Hunza now, I'll feel that I have reached the peak of my existence."

Hunza, a remote state in West Pakistan since 1947, has been an independent kingdom and a land of mystery for more than two thousand years. People refer to it as "Shangri-La," as the "Valley of Eternal Youth." Some speak of it as "a lost paradise." No matter what it is called, the ones who were lucky to visit it returned with fantastic stories about this fascinating land.

In spite of being part of Pakistan, Hunza has kept its independence and is ruled by a royal family. His Highness Mohammed Jamal Khan, the Mir, is the ruler of Hunza. With its unique position, bordering on China, Russia, Kashmir, Afghanistan, and India, Hunza occupies a place of great political importance. Until recently it has been closed to visitors and tourists, and only a few have managed to enter. A special entry permit was required, and it took me almost a year of red tape to get one. Even the president of Pakistan had to extend a helping hand to issue my entry to Hunza. And, of course, the Mir's personal invitation helped to speed it up.

Hunza has a population of over 30,000 people. In a very real sense the story of the Hunza people is the story of active, happy people. They take great pride in their continuous progress. Entering the valley, you catch the mood of happiness and peace that is ever-present among the residents of this fine community.

No matter where you appear, you are greeted with their usual "Saiaam." (It is the same as our "How do you do.") Soon one has a feeling of belonging to a community of the friendliest neighbors you've ever met.

The Hunzakuts say: "Health is the basic principle of happiness!" Thus, they have adopted the basic rules of health by following a simple diet, exercising daily, breathing rhythmically, relaxing, and formulating a positive philosophy.

The Hunza people live to a ripe old age in almost perfect mental and physical health. Cancer or heart disease do not kill them in the prime of their lives. They are able to retain their youthful appearance and partake in daily activities no matter how old they are. Young men play games with older men, and it doesn't seem to bother anybody.

The type of food they eat and have eaten for centuries, the way they cook and prepare their meals, the water they drink— all have something to do with their remarkable health, vigor, and endurance. Walking is part of their way of life. Their homes and gardens are on hilly locations, as is most of their land; thus walking is a habit and a necessity. The hard physical labor of working is another means of daily exercise.

The men mix work with exercise and pleasure. They take time off from their work during the day to participate in games and dances, and then return to the fields to resume their jobs. One of the reasons the men can walk long distance, exercise, and play games, and then return to work without a sign of fatigue is their ability to relax every muscle and nerve in their bodies. This protects the muscles from overwork and is a part of the yoga regime discussed in a later chapter.

Their ability to live in peace and brotherhood has given them peace of mind. They meditate and pray regularly. Belonging to the Muslim religion, some of them pray five times a day, in the privacy of their homes or in little mosques built in every village throughout the land. They seem to have an undying faith in God, and fear is foreign to them.

"There is no need for the body to get sick under the strain of life, or for the mind to shatter under tension, or the heart to fail, because it is driven beyond its strength," the Mir has said to me. It is obvious that the Hunza way of life is one of mental and spiritual balance. Without strong bodies, however, these people would not possess their great inner strength.

As I have observed, the people of Hunza do not consciously follow any special diet, or talk about it. Nor are they concerned about their weight. In fact, there is no obesity. Men and women are slim. Women walk with a light glide, and in spite of living in complete isolation, they seem to be very feminine and aware of their looks. They love to dress up and to wear jewelry. I couldn't help but notice their beautiful complexions.

The women have no time for coffee klatshces. Each day is full and planned. I have seen women of eighty or older doing physical chores and afterwards walking up 1,200-foot pathways to their homes without showing signs of fatigue. An aged couple working for the Mir as gardeners take this walk a few times every day. They had the opportunity to live on the palace grounds, but their choice was the house high up in the hills.

Women are not concerned with their calendar age. No one is judged by a calendar, and there is no fear that time is passing away. To their way of thinking one is as old as one looks, or as one feels, or as one behaves. Old age is not looked upon with dread; on the contrary, the young people look up to their elders, realizing they have accumulated years of valuable experience.

Raising a family is considered a sacred obligation. The same goes for marriage. It is not taken lightly, and a divorce is foreign in this tiny land of happy people. Naturally, the children are assigned work to do and they have to assume responsibilities at an early age. They play an important role in the household, and from childhood on, respect for their elders, whether relatives, parents, or neighbors, has been instilled in them. The child grows in a happy yet strict atmosphere, and accepts his place in society with dignity and understanding.

The parents have confidence that their children will do no wrong, and on many occasions let them use their own judgment. I had an interesting experience while I was there. My guide was an eight-year-old boy. As we walked down the hill, hand-in-hand, a beautiful woman walked up the hill. She carried a bundle on her shoulders. Her smile was radiant. The boy and she exchanged the greeting of "Salaam."

The boy quietly said: "That was my mother coming home from the fields. We live up this hill." As he uttered these words, there was pride and assurance in his voice. He knew he belonged to a family who loved him dearly. "She is beautiful, your mother!" I remarked. "Oh, yes, I know!" Still a child, he was a full grown man in his attitude.

How many mothers would walk by seeing their youngster with a complete stranger and not stop to query where he was going and when he would be home? She had confidence that her son could do no wrong, and she expected him to behave properly without her interference. Self-assurance, self-confidence, and faith were among the many lessons I learned in the land of Hunza

Man strives to overcome the obstacles that stand in the way of his happiness and peace of mind—and in the process pushes himself to exhaustion without giving much thought to his health. He forgets that health comes first, since without health man can hardly find happiness in wealth.

In the tiny land of Hunza, where there is no human disease, no animal disease, no plant disease and where there is no crime, no juvenile delinquency, no divorces—and obviously no police force or jails, as no one needs them—one has to stop to think. All the inspiring messages of the great religious texts are demonstrated here by these simple, God-loving people. Should not this give us a clue to finding mutual understanding and a way to operate together for the benefit of all?

Nevertheless, Hunza was not always the peaceful valley that it is today. Once, the clangorous sounds of battle echoed through the mountain passes. Apparently, the Hunzakuts are descendants of three soldiers from Alexander the Great's army. While his forces were campaigning at the Oxus River, these young men married beautiful Persian maidens, and when the army turned south, the soldiers, weary of battle, deserted. In their search for peace and freedom, they discovered this wondrous valley and settled there. Ironically enough, the Hunzakuts, in order to keep their valley safe from invaders were forced to become as fierce and barbaric as their foes. Even the armies of Genghis Khan failed to conquer them.

The difficulty of the road to Hunza, which still exists today, proved to be their most valuable weapon. For centuries this road, a scant 24-inch pathway which threads itself over and across the towering precipices of the Himalayas, was the main highway between Kashgar, in Sinkiang, and Kashmir.

At first, the Hunzakuts used their force to protect the valley, but as years went on, it became their habit to destroy anything and anybody who came near their territory. Even peaceful neighbors suffered from their cruelties. Chinese traders agreed to pay tribute to them so that they could cross the mountains with their caravans laden with silks, tea and porcelain, on their way to India, and then return to Cathay with spices, jewels, ivory and gold.

Naturally, the Hunzakuts accepted rich bribes from the traders, promising to let them through, but seldom kept their word. As they saw the Chinese packtrains, they would scale the high peaks and hurl huge boulders down upon the road, sending the helpless caravans into dizzying chasms hundreds of feet below. Then at their leisure, with no merchant left alive, they would recover their booty.

It was not until the grandfather of the present Mir, Sir Mohammed Nazim Khan, became ruler of Hunza that the promise of peace was made and upheld. And the same peace has now reigned throughout the land for over eighty years. Their new ruler succeeded in persuading his people to settle down to a peaceful agricultural occupation, and after a while the wild mountain slopes were turned into magnificent gardens.

The Hunzakuts have learned their lesson. Somewhere in the distant past, they must have realized that fighting and killing are the negative aspects of life—that there are many other values in life which they were missing. Within a span of a few years they became a peaceful group of people. Their record of good health is amazing and it seems to pervade all other aspects of their life. But the level of their spiritual development should not be overlooked. They are faithful to God's teachings and live their religion every wakeful moment. H.R.H. Karim Aga Khan is their spiritual leader and they truly love and respect him.

Having the good fortune to stay at the palace as the guest of the royal family, I was able to see so much. Their hospitality exceeded all expectation. The influence of England and its customs prevailed here at the palace household. It was unique, perfect. During the meals a parade of splendid dishes were served by the three butlers in native uniforms in an atmosphere of unmatched elegance. And amidst all of this was Her Highness the Rani (the Queen), so delicate, so gentle, so humble, and so beautiful. At the head of the table she was like a shining candle, like a life force formed by creation guarding her shrine. I could feel the boundless strength of an eternal energy, in spite of her fragile appearance.

And the six princesses, daughters of the royal family, all were beautiful, resembling their mother, yet every one had a different personality. Slender and so very graceful they were endowed with a limitless vitality.

And then there were three young sons, the princes, including the crown prince, Ghazanfar Khan, who will take the throne when his father retires. He had a strong face, a sense of responsibility behind his child-like look. (He was then sixteen years old.) The two other brothers also looked relaxed and comfortable in the presence of their royal parents and strangers.

Prince Ayash, the Mir's brother, was a noble gentleman with

a broad smile and a gentle voice, always ready to help.

The palace, a two story structure of mixed architecture—oriental in design with a modern flavor—was a pleasant place built of hand-hewn Hunza granite. And the richly landscaped garden filled the whole palace with an exotic fragrance. And at the end of the valley there was the mountain wall of the Himalayas protecting this tiny kindgom from all evils.

There is no light of any kind available in Hunza. Even candle or kerosine would be too expensive to import, so people have to go to bed early and rise early. Since it has become a habit, no one resents it. At the palace a small Diesel engine supplies light for two hours during the evening meal, but at ten everyone retires, as life begins again at four o'clock in the morning. The prayer man, with a piercing sound which can be heard all over the valley, wakes the people up, calling them to pray before they start their chores of the day. And the same happens when the sun goes down; he calls them to pray, and afterwards to go to rest. These people are very religious, but they are not fanatics. They usually pray in silent meditation.

Even the Mir himself comes to the cemetery, and at the tomb of his beloved grandfather spends hours reading the Koran in a low voice, chanting from the sacred book, in surroundings of absolute peace. He knows that the past has gone forever, as far as they are concerned, and that these majestic mountains are the only witness of the cruelties his ancestors practiced.

Dr. Robert C. McCarrison, an English surgeon who took up the study of diseases of the peoples of Asia, after he met up with the Hunzakuts, writes about them: "My own experience provides an example of a race unsurpassed in perfection of physique and in freedom from disease in general. I refer to the people of the State of Hunza. Amongst these people the span of life is extraordinarily long. . . . During the period of my association with these people, I never saw a case of asthenic dyspepsia, of gastric or duodenal ulcer, or appendicitis, of mucous colitis, or cancer. . . . Among these people the abdomen oversensitive to nerve impressions, to fatigue, anxiety or cold was unkown."

In an article written by Dr. McCarrison in 1926, he mentions some of the other races, inhabitants of the Himalayan Mountains, who were quite "of fine physical development and power of endurance, but by no means even compare with the Hunzakuts."

The Hunzakuts do not contaminate their plants or their soil. Their food is pure and fresh. They eat mainly grains, leafy vegetables, fruits, dairy products and some meat.

They also exercise faithfully and walk a great deal, since they live mostly up in the hills. They also play various games, such as volleyball, archery, tennis, and polo. Some riding is done, too. All these games are played in addition to their daily activities in the fields. These people are very active; there is no time for idleness, and no time to grow old.

They have learned to live in peace and harmony, and they respect each other. They have great faith in God. Their spiritual awareness never ceased to amaze me. To them religion is something that is not only read about, or preached about, but a way of life. . . .

Which is greater, worldly wealth that is here today and gone tomorrow or the wealth of divine love that God has bestowed upon these people? Divine love is the magnet that draws all good! The wealth of divine love has met every need of man!

A group that draws together automatically through conscious or unconscious affinity of purpose finds that there is no overlapping of function, no competition, only a thorough conviction that no one can achieve contentment unless everyone achieves it.

These people are bound together in the common love that is truly the mother of humanity—the only torch that can lead the way to peace.

THE HUNZA DIET

LUNCH
Salad—consisting of fresh vegetables, cut up. Apricot oil and grape vinegar served separately as a dressing.
Cheese
Chapatti
A beverage—milk or lassi, or yogurt.

DINNER
A vegetable stew with millet, barley, or rice added to it.
Chapatti
A dessert or fresh fruit.

The Hunza people eat two meals a day. There isn't enough food for them to partake of more meals. But in between the meals and in the morning they drink water which they call "Glacier Milk," as it is of a grayish color. It comes from the melting snow from the glaciers, and brings the rich minerals with it. They are very lucky. The daily supply of fresh minerals nourishes their bodies, and apparently the body requires a great amount of minerals to be well. These minerals cannot be stored in the body, a fresh supply every day is essential.

Recently, I lectured at San Diego College, in National City in California, discussing the Hunza people and their health habits. After the program, Doctor C.S. Hansen came to meet me, to tell me that research is being conducted to determine the value of minerals in the human body, and that important findings might soon be revealed to the public.

The water which is served at the palace in Hunza comes directly from the glaciers and is full of sand which one feels under the teeth. But it tastes very good, so one gets used to it in no time at all. However, for the guests at the palace, if they prefer, the water is filtered and served clear. Obviously, the muddy water has more nutritional value—if one can overlook the sand.

Bread—Chapatti

Since the Hunzakuts have no mechanized farm equipment, all grains are harvested by hand. After being threshed, the grain is stored in a dry place, ready to be ground into flour as it is needed. The grain is ground in an ancient gristmill, operated by water from the irrigation system. By this method, the flour retains all of the natural nutrients found in wheat, including the bran and wheat germ.

Out of this flour "chapattis" are baked over an open fire by using a flat rock or a piece of metal. Chapattis are an example of the unleavened "staff of life" that is referred to in our Bible. The preparation of chapattis is quite complicated, an art that has been handed down from mother to daughter for centuries. They are made from wheat, barley, buckwheat, or millet; occasionally the flours are mixed together and baked in several shapes, small or large, according to the occasion.

This Hunza bread is wholesome, unrefined, maybe even coarse, but full of good nourishment. The part of the grain from which the new plant grows is called the germ. This germ is actually the most nourishing portion of the grain. The outer covering of the grain is known as bran. This gives the flour a brownish coloring. The Hunza people don't eat white flour; they have never seen it or tasted it. So by leaving in the germ and the bran, they make their flour full of excellent nourishment. This germ is known to us as "wheat germ" which supplies Vitamin E. It is also the part of the grain which seems to assist the sexual powers of the animal who eats it, according to H. A. Mattill, M.D., who conducted an experiment and reported it in the *American Journal of Physiology* as far back as 1927. And then Dr. Evan Shute, of Canada, reported, in the *Urological and Cutaneous Review*, Volume 48, 1944, of using vitamin E extensively in therapy for productive disorders.

Hunza bread consists of all the nutrients of the grain. Maybe it accounts for the Hunzakuts' strong nerves and vigor into old age, as well as for the fact that their men are capable of fathering children at very old ages. Having lived for generations on sturdy brown bread, white bread doesn't appeal to them. Besides, course brown bread is chewy and exercises the gums.

Milk

Milk is a complete food. In Hunza it is used in various ways. The cream is separated and made into ghee, a sort of butter. Cottage cheese is made from the remains, and is a vital source of protein in their diet. Most of these products are made from goat's milk. Fresh, raw milk is nourishing and rich in protein. The Hunzakuts have no pasteurization system and have to drink the raw milk.

Vegetables

Vegetables play a great part in the Hunzakuts' diet, and since they don't cook too much, heat doesn't destroy the valuable nutrients stored in the plant. Every food consists of minerals, vitamins, enzymes and proteins, and when its values are diminished by extreme heat, there is little left to nourish our bodies.

The Hunzakuts don't grow too many vegetables, due to lack of tillable soil, but what they have has obviously been a wise choice. They grow leafy vegetables, such as spinach and lettuce, and cucumbers, radishes, carrots, turnips, and potatoes and a variety of herbs, which are used in cooking and also in beverages.

Cooking is done in covered vessels over a very low fire. If the vegetables are cooked in water, this liquid is served with them. Nothing is discarded or thrown away. All the minerals, such as phosphorus, calcium, iron, iodine, and many other valuable nutrients are consumed as food available in these tasty vegetables.

In Hunza, vegetables come directly from the gardens; they are fresh, and they are not sprayed with any chemicals, as it is forbidden by law to attempt to spray gardens. These vegetables and fruits can be eaten raw with the skin, which contains many valuable mineral salts, most of which are lost in soaking, vigorous scrubbing, peeling, and cooking.

Fruits

Apples, pears, peaches, mulberries, black and red cherries, and grapes are grown in moderate quantities. The Hunzas' favorite fruit is apricot. Apricots are eaten raw in summer and sun-dried for the winter. The Hunzas have learned to extract from the kernel of the apricot a very rich oil which they use for cooking, salad dressing, even as a cosmetic on their skins and hair.

We always hear that a diet should be balanced and complete—consisting of proteins, carbohydrates, fats, minerals, vitamins, water, and oxygen. I sometimes wonder whether the Hunzakuts were aware of this factor, but maybe by instinct they realized that food without fat doesn't taste good, that something is lacking. A long search to find fat in some of their foods led them to discover it in the seed of the apricot. It is not simple to prepare, but nothing seems too much for them when it means their good health and survival. Since they don't eat pork, being Moslems, and very little other animal fat is available, they have no other choice but to produce their apricot oil. The results prove worthwhile, as it tastes delicious, it enriches the flavor of the food, and is supposed to be rich in polyunsaturated fats. The freedom from circulatory disease, heart attacks, and strokes that the Hunzakuts enjoy makes one wonder. . . .

Meat

The Hunza people are not vegetarians, but they eat very little meat and it is served only on special occasions. And when they cook it, it is prepared in a form of a stew, and small portions are dished out. Chickens until recently were not allowed to be brought in, for fear they would destroy the crops by pecking the seeds. Recently this has changed, and you can find a few chickens wandering around. Children play with them, since there are no dogs or cats, for lack of food to feed an extra animal. The chickens take the place of a family pet. Then, of course, the eggs have enriched the diet! An additional supply of proteins is a great luxury.

Occasionally, these people run out of food at the end of the winter season. Until the new crop is available, they have practically nothing to eat, and water has to suffice. Apparently it nourishes them well, and they easily survive the period of near-starvation. We would call it "fasting," a method which has been adopted by a number of sanatoriums and clinics all over Europe, especially in Switzerland and Germany.

Hippocrates, the father of medicine, suggested fasts up to

seven days and stated: "Hunger reacts in the nature of man with great power and can be considered the means that leads to recovery from disease." He was a great believer in fasting and also in a natural way of eating, in exercising, and in morning walks. He said, "Your food should be your medicine."

The Hunza palace cuisine would please the most critical gourmet, and I enjoyed many exotic, delicious new dishes while I was there. Most of the meals were served formally, but the buffet dinners served from time to time, with their natural informality, were very pleasant.

The Hunzakuts work very hard from sunrise to sunset, six days a week, and use a tremendous amount of physical energy. Nevertheless, they eat little and do very well on their frugal diet, compared to the variety and quantity of foods the average American thinks he needs each day to survive. My housekeeper, a wonderful person, is quite argumentative when it comes to meat. She claims that without eating meat at least twice a day, she doesn't have physical strength to work. I don't intend to convince her, but I have seen and lived with the Hunza people. Excess weight is unusual among them. They enjoy good teeth, sturdy bone structure, good eyesight, normal digestion, and sound hearts. A general condition of perfect health is the rule rather than the exception in Hunza. So who can argue with them?

Above all the Hunzakuts demonstrate that a peaceful life can be enjoyed. People can shake off a heritage of greed, jealousy, and cravings for power. The Hunzakuts have demonstrated that love and a spiritually inspired life brings happiness. When we truly learn to understand each other, to fulfill the precepts of brotherly love and live a simple life, then we, too, will be able to find peace within ourselves.

Captured by the spell of the whole valley, the friendly and joyous people, I saw everything in a new light. Why can't we learn that the readiness to enjoy life is no shallow childishness but the deep source of blessed living?

HUNZA RECIPES

The following recipes were given to me by the gracious Rani who taught me how to cook the Hunza way. Of course, I've more or less adapted certain recipes to include nutritional products and natural ingredients obtainable in our own country.

Kamali—Plain Chapatti

(BASIC RECIPE)

2 cups whole wheat flour (stone ground)
½ teaspoon vegetable salt or sea salt
¾ to 1 cup water

Blend flour and salt together. Stir in just enough water to make a very stiff dough. Knead dough on a lightly floured surface until smooth and elastic. Cover with a wet cloth: set aside for 30 minutes. Break the dough into one inch balls, and roll out into very thin rounds, about 8 inches in diameter. Bake for 10 minutes on a hot, lightly greased griddle over low heat; turn often. It makes 20 chapattis.

Kalchar—Small Chapattis

2 cups of whole wheat flour
(stone ground)
⅛ lb. of margarine (rich in un-
saturated fatty acid)
½ cup buttermilk
½ teaspoon mineral sea salt

Mix margarine with flour, then blend milk in a little at a time.

Variations:

1. Chapattis on grill—thin and crisp.
   Roll dough paper thin and cook on pre-heated griddle. It is
   excellent with salads or soups. Can be kept in an airtight
   container and it will remain crisp for future use.

2. Roll dough about ¾″ thick and cut out like small biscuits. Bake
   in oven in greased pan. Pre-heat oven to 350° then turn
   down to 250° and bake until done.

The Hunza stone-ground flour contains more bran than our
usual flour. Therefore, the consistency might be different and it
is advisable to add some bran flour to the mixture. Also they do
not use salt, as their food is full of natural minerals. Our taste
requires flavoring of food. We suggest using sea salt or vegetable salt.

Piti-Chapatti

(BASIC RECIPE)

> 2 cups whole wheat flour (stone
>   ground)
> ¾ cup milk and luke warm water
>   (half-and-half to equal the
>   ¾ measurement)
> ½ teaspoon vegetable salt
> ¼ cup saf-flower oil

Mix flour with milk and water, add oil and salt. Make into a dough and roll out to a ½-inch thick loaf and bake in a 350° oven (pre-heated). Mix dough thoroghly, stirring mixture by hand. The longer you stir the dough, the more you develop the gluten in the flour and the more elastic it will become and the lighter the bread will be.

Cheese Chapatti

> ½ cup whole wheat flour
> 1½ cups buckwheat flour
> ½ teaspoon baking power
> ½ teaspoon vegetable salt
> 3¼ cups buttermilk
> 2 eggs
> 2 tablespoons sweet butter or
>   preferably saf-flower oil

Sift flour and then add salt and baking powder. Pour into a bowl, add buttermilk and melted butter or saf-flower oil, beat egg yolks and add . . . then blend dry ingredients and beat the batter until it is smooth and elastic . . . add the stiffly beaten whites of the eggs. Bake chapattis on a medium hot griddle following customary rules. Makes 8 large chapattis.

Filling:

Blend 2 cups of cottage cheese with buttermilk until smooth. add vegetable salt to taste. Lay out one chapatti and spread cheese all over, cover with another and repeat till all are used. Let stand for 2 hours then cut like a cake and serve.

Millet Bread

> *1 cup millet flour*
> *1 cup grated golden carrots*
> *1 tablespoon honey*
> *1 tablespoon vegetable salt*
> *2 tablespoons corn-oil*
> *2 eggs*

Combine in bowl: Millet flour, carrots, oil, honey and salt. Mix well, then stir ¾ cup of boiling hot water into the mixture. Beat the egg yolks well adding 2 tablespoons of cold water, continue to beat and then add to the mixture. Fold in stiffly beaten whites of eggs and bake in hot, oiled pan at 350° for about 40 minutes.

Millet Casserole

1 cup hulled millet
½ cup diced carrots
½ cup diced green fresh peppers
1 cup fresh mushrooms (cut)
2 tablespoons saf-flower oil
1 teaspoon vegetable salt
¼ teaspoon salad herbs
¼ cup whole almonds

Heat the oil in a heavy skillet, stir the millet and brown slightly. Add the chopped vegetables . . . vegetable salt, and stir for three minutes. Put the mixture into a covered saucepan adding enough water to cover about one inch above the millet . . . add almonds and cook over low heat for 15 minutes, then continue for a while in a double boiler . . . until tender . . . (6 servings).

Millet—Hulled

½ cup hulled millet
1 cup water
1 cup milk
  dried apricots—(soaked in
  bottled water overnight, just
  enough to cover the fruit)
½ teaspoon vegetable salt

Heat water and milk in top part of double boiler . . . add millet and steam over boiling water for 30 minutes or until millet is tender. Serve hot . . . add apricots and liquid . . . (sunflower seed meal and almond meal or ground nuts can be added). Millet is very nourishing and rich in proteins . . . for a quick breakfast, prepare in double boiler the night before. (4 to 6 servings.)

The Hunzas use millet frequently, serving with dried apricots or fresh in season. They don't use any sweetening, but their fruit has an entirely different taste . . . if you prefer it sweet, honey is advisable.

Whole Buckwheat Groats

1 cup whole buckwheat groats
*2 cups of water**
1 teaspoon vegetable salt
2 tablespoons of saf-flower oil
1 egg

Heat the oil in a heavy skillet, stir in the buckwheat mixed priorly with the beaten whole egg. Add the vegetable salt and brown slightly, keeping it stirred with a spoon. Finally, add the water, bring to a boil, then reduce the heat. Cover tightly and let cook until all liquid is absorbed. It must never be mushy. Every grain should be separate. (6 servings.)

*Instead of the water you can use vegetable broth in the form of a powder. (The Health Food Stores have a variety of vegetable broth brands.) Pour a cup of hot water over a teaspoon of the powder. It makes a delicious soup and can also be used instead of water in the buckwheat groats.

Hunza Mint Soup

To any broth such as lamb, beef or chicken, the addition of a tablespoon of chopped mint per serving will greatly improve the flavor. Also, blend in some buckwheat groats.

Hunza Lamb Stew

> 2 *pounds of lamb shoulders*
> 1 *quart of water*
> 1 *tablespoon vegetable salt*
> 3 *small carrots—sliced*
> 2 *stalks of celery—diced parsley, bay leaf and sprig dried thyme, tied together in a bundle*
> 1 *tablespoon lemon juice*
> 10 *small onions peeled (onions can be omitted)*
> ¼ *lb. mushrooms, sliced*
> 2½ *tablespoons saf-flower oil*
> 1 *cup of Yogurt*

Cut lamb into small pieces, cover with water, bring to boil, then skim off all excess fat . . . add the vegetables and the bundle of herbs. Cover with a lid and cook over slow heat for about 30 minutes, or until the meat is tender.

Sautée the mushrooms in oil in a separate pan for about 5 to 10 minutes. Add the mushrooms to the meat, there should be sufficient liquid (about 3 cups) in the stew . . . add vegetable salt . . . beat the Yogurt with 1 tablespoon lemon juice and pour in some of the hot gravy, mixing it briskly. Then add to the meat . . . cook for a few minutes below boiling point—always cook over low heat—before serving sprinkle with parsley. (6 servings.)

Hunza Golden Brown Lamb Pillau

1 pound of brown rice
2 teaspoons vegetable salt
   Enough water to cover rice
1 lb. of carrots
½ cup of saf-flower oil
2 pounds of meat (lamb)
2 large onions (could be
   omitted)

Cut onions finely and brown in oil. Blend in carrots cut into squares. Keep stirring for about 10 minutes over low heat . . . add meat cut up into fairly small pieces and cover with water. Let it cook until the meat is done. Keep it covered all the time . . . take out meat only, strain soaked rice and add to the soup. After ½ hour, add the pre-cooked meat and cook a little longer, covered with a lid.

Hunza Cutlets

(BASIC RECIPE)

1 pound of minced meat—beef,
* lamb* or veal, but no pork*
1 cup of water
1 egg
1 teaspoon vegetable salt

Mix meat well with the water. Beat the egg yolk and blend with the meat. Add the vegatable salt. Mix well. Beat stiffly the white of the egg, and blend with the meat . . . makes three large cutlets or four smaller ones . . . pre-heat the skillet, place cutlets in without fat, cover with the lid and cook over low heat for 5 minutes. Pour off the excess fat and continue to cook still over low heat, turning the cutlets, browning them on both sides. After a while pour off some more fat. The meat should not get the excess fat at any time. (Serve hot.)

*The Hunzas use mostly lamb.

Creamed Spinach

Use 2 pounds of new spinach. Wash it in several waters until it is free of sand. Lift from water with hands and place in a well covered saucepan without adding water. The moisture is sufficient. Cover and simmer over low heat for about five minutes . . . or until it is tender . . . drain well . . . let it cool off and chop it fine, using a board and a knife, or in a blender. Pour 2 tablespoons of saf-flower oil into a skillet and simmer spinach for a few minutes, just to heat it through . . . season with vegetable salt to taste . . . remove from the heat . . . stir in slowly one cup of Yogurt and ¼ lb. of ground almonds. Sprinkle with fresh chopped parsley. (4 servings.)

Hunza Spinach in Chapattis

Prepare spinach by the same recipe as above . . . add 1 cup chopped mushrooms sauteed in 2 tablespoons of saf-flower oil. Blend with spinach. Make thin chapattis (see recipe, page 28), or use a ready mix* . . . place a large tablespoon of the mixture on each chapatti, roll them and sprinkle with grated raw tillamook cheese, or place a slice of cheese on top . . . then broil** them for a few minutes until the cheese is melted.

*Whole wheat stone ground ready mix is available in your favorite Health Food Store, and your market.

**An electric stainless steel low temperature skillet can be used instead of a broiler, keep lid-covered at all times.

Hunza Eggs in Spinach

Fill a buttered baking dish with creamed spinach (see Creamed Spinach recipe). Press hollows in the spinach with a large spoon. Break one egg into each hollow. Season with vegetable salt or seasoning salt . . . place the dish into a pan of hot water in an oven of about 325° for about 10 minutes (until the eggs are firm), sprinkle with grated raw tillamook cheese and chopped parsley, keep for another minute in the oven until the cheese is melted, add chopped parsley before serving. (4 servings.)

This dish can be baked in an electric skillet.

Hunza Spinach Curry With Meat

2 pounds spinach, wash, and drain. Chop it fine and let it stay for a while. Shortly before serving warm the spinach including the juice in a double boiler . . . adding 1 teaspoon vegetable salt, 2 teaspoons curry powder . . . cook slowly over low heat for about 5 minutes . . . add 2 tablespoons of saf-flower oil and ¼ lb ground almonds . . . mix well.

In a saucepan filled with water, place 2 lbs. of finely cut pieces of lamb (shanks). Add 2 carrots (quartered), 3 stalks of celery (cut in 1″ pieces), 2 onions (quartered). Cover with a lid and cook over low heat . . . when meat is practically done and very little water is left, take out the vegetables which were added for taste only, but are not used. Now blend in the spinach curry and serve hot. (6 servings.)

Grape Vinegar

Wash grapes well and place in a wooden bowl for seven days. Mash grapes with hands, then strain through a cheese cloth. Place the juice in a glass bottle and seal well. Keep for 40 days before using.

Grape Wine

Use same method as preparing vinegar, but keep bottles in a cool place for 90 days. When the wine is sweet it is ready.

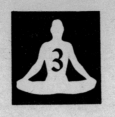

Yoga, the Art of Living

Possibly no other science is more misunderstood than the science of Yoga.

Some of the Hindus from India who visit the Western countries are often not too well equipped to teach or represent Yoga philosophy, which actually should be considered as a way of life. But some of these people lack the true Yogic idealism, the necessary spiritual evolution. Even in India, Yoga until recently has been often misrepresented, and thus misunderstood, and followed by only a handful of people.

So often when hearing of a Yogi, the teacher or guru (master), one pictures a man with matted locks and unkempt beard, untidy in appearance. It is assumed that such a man eats practically nothing, survives on herbs and water and lives in some remote cave or on top of a mountain.

Some Yogis who have come to this country demonstrated quite unusual things, such as chewing glass and digesting it; drinking nitric acid, which is known to be a strong poison, with no affect on their health; levitating from the ground while meditating; indulging in predictions; or performing many other things foreign to our experience. None of these things has anything to do with Yoga. In fact, the very complicated postures they assume, which could be considered physical acrobatics, and the prolonged retention of breath—these are not the purpose of yoga.

Maybe you heard of a man who lived in Hollywood. He called himself a Yogi. At his own request he was placed in a coffin and buried alive. Several days later, the coffin was dug out and he was found to be in perfect health. This feat can be accomplished by extraordinary breathing skill. The same technique is used when sitting on a bed of nails, feeling no pain and having no scars left afterwards. But this is not necessary to become a good student of Yoga. On the contrary, these demonstrations make people shy away from real Yoga practices.

Here is another example of how much harm the wrong publicity about Yoga can do. A reporter of the Associated Press from New Delhi, India, reported a story about a well-known yogi, L.S. Rao, who claimed that he would demonstrate to a select group who were willing to pay the money that he could walk on water. Rao sank like a rock in the specially made tank.

As in every step of Yoga, the deep rhythmic breathing has a significant bearing on the mind, and by the control of breath it is possible to enjoy a longer life, too. But the breathing is an aid to meditation and spiritual unfoldment and must not be turned into a fetish, or used as a means for gaining control over physical laws.

Yoga must not be taken for a Hindu dogma. It is not a religion by itself. The literal meaning of the term "Yoga" is "union." The Bagha Va Gita (a part of orthodox Hindu scripture, and considered by many Westerners the most important of all Hindu philosophical and religious books) says, "Efficiency in action is Yoga." Anyway we can make this statement with assurance that yoga is primarily a *way of life*, facing the *reality of life*, and by no means a running away from *life* or the *world*.

The world is not bad in itself; it is the slavery of man to his senses that is bad. A positive attachment is not a very bad thing. It is the physical part of it, the selfish possessiveness, which negates true love. "Attachment" to principles, to noble values, could not be rated as something bad. "Action sculptures your life; action sculptures the world. You practice the art of action when you act to bring the good into visibility." (From *The Art of Living*, by Wilfred A. Peterson.)

The world of senses, which we feel and see, enjoy and suffer from, is not the only reality. There is something else which is beyond our reach, beyond all that is apparent. Life is not entirely matterbound. Something is greater than temporal values. It is imperative to acquire a degree of control over one's mind and not be carried away by our likes and dislikes, or unforseen setbacks.

To control one's thinking and moods is very important. You shouldn't get elated over material gains, which usually don't last too long, or plunge into a negative state of depression due to a loss or suffering. Here the role of discrimination comes into play. It is one of the initial steps in Yoga. One's sufferings are an outcome of the association of one's body and mind, one's individuality, with a temporary state of existence. It is the body and the mind that act and enjoy and suffer. Yoga enables you to be guided by your conscience in your conduct and action. It is said that a twinge of conscience is a glimpse of God.

Man suffers because of a negative strain of sensual attachment to objects or individuals, an attachment that pertains to his physical and mental individuality. Man would therefore be in a much better position to perform his duties well if he trained himself to be a useful instrument for the working of the will of God—that is, performing action without any selfish motivation or any expectation of material gain as an exclusive objective of his action.

Of course, this requires a good deal of evolution in spiritual life. Efficiency, perseverance, initiative—these should be the guiding factors of one's active life. Only then can action be called Yoga. Thus, the real objective of Yoga is to keep the material interests of life within legitimate limits, and eliminate greed from one's life and from that of others.

A sense of oneness with God is Yoga. To what extent your devotion to God finds expression in your conduct, your attitude toward personal gain, and your outlook toward your fellow-beings is the yardstick of knowing your progress in the path of the Yoga of devotion.

God is not confined to one image. He is in every image and yet beyond all. If you expect Him to behave like a great earthly potentate and if you ascribe worldly virtues to His greatness, your concept of God is limited to the level of your evolution and is indicative of your characteristics. The moment you confine God to a form, you limit Him.

But one needs a symbol to approach Him, to have a concept to meditate upon and draw inspiration from. It is, however, a very open question as to how far a spiritual aspirant could benefit by being satisfied with limiting his concept of God to an apotheosis, even though it be that of a magnificent and virtuous householder.

"Action releases truth so it can inspire and regenerate; action releases ideas so they can bless and benefit." (From *The Art of Living*, by Wilfred A. Peterson.)

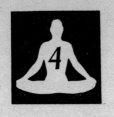

Yoga, and Its
Basic Principles

Physical fitness has become the talk of our century. Quite a lot has been said about it, but it is basically a plan, a method to keep your body conditioned to all circumstances—weather changes, extremes of temperature, high or sea-level altitude, various climates. It helps to build a strong resistance to accept the various changes without affecting your health. A physically fit person will usually endure strain better and have greater stamina than a person with an unfit body.

A healthy person can cope much better with nervous tension and ignore physical stress. A body is a delicate mechanism which will serve you well, as long as you treat it accordingly. Stop winding up your watch and it will stop working. A neglected body has no resistance and muscles begin sagging, blood circulation slows down, and age creeps in.

Yoga can teach you how to attain bodily poise, how to control your breath, and how to relax. It is based on the following principles:

1. Correct deep rhythmic breathing.
2. Exercise.
3. Relaxation.
4. Concentration.
5. Meditation.
6. Diet and nutrition.

By practicing Yoga daily, without fail, you will begin to function better; you will improve your posture, your voice, your eyesight, your eating habits, as well as promote the functioning of all your joints, limbs, muscles, and other parts of the body.

Everything we do, such as drinking, eating, sleeping, working, has a significance, and if we learn how to do these things properly, with moderation and tranquility, we shall be able to experience a fuller and healthier life.

A Tibetan aphorism defines Yoga as "An Art of Living enabling us to use every activity of the body, language, and spirit." In fact, a good Yoga work-out can open the door to a radiant, well-balanced, relaxed, and youthful future.

There are many branches of Yoga, but in this book we'll deal mainly with the physical Yoga, known as Hatha Yoga. It is a simple method, and can be practiced in our Western civilization with excellent results. It is an exact science based on scientific principles; it imparts to everyone who practices Yoga, definite practical knowledge, fine health, longevity, strength, and vitality.

Yoga is an ancient yet still unsurpassed science of living. In Yoga, relaxation is an art, breathing a science, and mental control a means of harmonizing body, mind, and spirit. It is recognized as a practical method to combat modern-day stress, strain and fatigue. Above all, practicing Yoga regularly will definitely perfect your physical health, lead you to mental discipline and to a better understanding of the spiritual aspect of man.

Yoga will teach you how to breathe correctly, how to relax, how and what to eat. It will help you to find harmony, peace, and true happiness. A clearer and calmer mind has an influence on your disposition, and suddenly you will feel that anger and stress have a grave influence on your health.

In the last few years much has been said about Yoga. Many new books have been published on this subject, articles written for national magazines. There is hardly a country where Yoga isn't being taught these days. But still, only a few are aware of what Yoga could do for every individual and consequently for the whole world.

Only the other day one of my students tried to arrange for a Yoga class at the condominion settlement were she lives with 1,200 other people. But she met with violent opposition. "Why do you want to bring a strange religion to our group?" she was asked. It proves once more how little is known about Yoga.

Too bad that Yoga is still taken as a religion, which it is not. It *is* a way of life, a method of physical fitness with high aspirations and deep aspects. There is scarcely a human being who would not benefit physically, morally, and spiritually by devoting even a little time to practicing Yoga.

Yoga teachings stand for truth, balance, rightness, a peaceful outlook and a benevolent attitude toward everybody, a progressive spirit and a deep faith in life and the deeper reality of which life is everywhere a manifestation. Yoga means simply to exert oneself, to discipline and apply oneself thoroughly to a given purpose, to practice, to study, to meditate and realize. It means all this and something more. And to *you* it will mean whatever you make out of it after you have given an honest trial practicing it.

Yoga is a path to wholeness, and it requires a wholesome outlook. Mind, body, and consciousness should be exerted as *one*. There are many branches of Yoga—the Karma Yoga, the Raja Yoga, the Gyana Yoga, the Bhakti Yoga, and the Laya Yoga—to suit everybody's temperament.

Karma Yoga is essentially the Yoga outlook and attitude that stresses *oneness* of life. Its basic commandments are truth and honesty. The *Gyana Yoga* aims at study and knowledge; *Bhakti Yoga* is the Yoga of devotion and selfless love; *Raja Yoga* is the science of mental control.

Raja Yoga has been divided into three more subdivisions known as *Mantra Yoga, Kundalini Yoga,* and *Hatha Yoga.* These are all various modes of practice.

But first we have to study Hatha Yoga to build our body and health, since the studies of the higher steps of Yoga need the foundation of a sound body and a sound mind. The word Hatha is composed of the syllables *ha* and *tha*, which mean ha (sun) and tha (moon). Hatha Yoga enfolds many aspects: *pranayama,* a variety of *deep breathing exercises; asanas,* or postures; *relaxation;* and *meditation.*

Yoga way of life does not interfere with any religion or faith and can be practiced by anyone who is sincere and willing to search for the truth. It holds the answer to many problems and a little effort can bring much in return!

As every science has its own method of investigation, so also the science of Yoga has its own method and declares that truth can be experienced. It is essential for a Yoga student to be patient, for many things will sound vague and strange at first; however, as he or she makes progress in learning more about the Yoga philosophy, it begins to make sense. The aim of it is to achieve truth wherein the individual soul identifies itself with the supreme soul or God. Thus it brings hope to the unhappy person, strength to the weak, and knowledge to the ignorant. In fact, Yoga is the secret key that unlocks the realm to deep abiding peace.

Yoga is primarily concerned with the inner being of man. If your spiritual practices enable you to attain a measure of mental purity, if your heart becomes more expansive and your outlook free from bias, if you are able to forgive those who harm you or hurt you, if you lose your temper only once in a while, instead of regularly, you have progressed on the path of Yoga.

DEEP RHYTHMIC BREATHING

We have learned that Hatha Yoga is a system of self-culture designed to attain harmonious development of the body, mind, intellect, and soul. We have also learned that what man needs to perfect himself lies within himself. That man is the "master" of his own doings.

Because of our living habits, breathing has become, among civilized people, more or less impaired. Of course, we breathe all the time, because we couldn't live without air. But our way of breathing is known as *shallow breathing*, from the chest, absorbing only a limited amount of oxygen, not sufficient for the lungs to work to full capacity. A short breath uses only a small part of the pulmonary capacity, and it doesn't ventilate the lungs properly, so that only a few of the air cells are functioning; thus the greater part of the lungs remain unused.

We'll all agree that one can live without food for days, but not without air. So *breath is the living force*. The Yogis became aware of this thousands of years ago, and the Western world is finally beginning to recognize its remarkable benefits. The Yogis call breath *prana*, a substance in the air which can be found in all things having life. We absorb prana from the food we eat, the water we drink, and the air we breathe. In fact, the whole body is controlled by the force of *prana*. Prana is a Sanskrit word symbolizing *universal energy*—life itself.

The control of prana opens the door to almost unlimited power. Yogis use this prana consciously for awakening the dormant spiritual force in man. They believe that between prana and the mind there exists an unexplainable relationship. No wonder that they above all stress the importance of proper breathing to maintain perfect health and vitality. Thus, the Yogis' theory is that the bodily postures combined with deep rhythmic breathing work to greater advantage when they are done together.

In spite of the fact that fresh air and correct habits of breathing are among the most valuable privileges of humanity, the majority of people have only a slight conception of their importance. Through the special deep rhythmic breathing we are able to store some oxygen in the solar plexus, the seat of vital energy in the body, which we need to keep in reserve for the time when our physical and mental health calls on these reserves.

Now, let's observe the way the majority of people do their breathing—mostly through the mouth. In this case the air comes directly through the throat into the bronchial tubes without being filtered or properly warmed up. The difference of temperature might cause a shock to the organs. It is possible that this cold air reaching the vital organs might be the cause for a bad cold or some other discomfort.

The connection between life and breatn is very close and breathing is the most essential biological function of the body. The Yogis were of an opinion that short breathing might shorten our lives, while the deeper inhalation might prolong life expectancy. Civilized man has forgotten the age-old system of rhythmical breathing because he doesn't understand the significance of all the wonderful and practical benefits derived from it.

Primitive man didn't need to learn how to breathe properly, since the physical conditions of his existence made him a good breather instinctively. He was closer to nature, and worked physically much harder. A child also is a natural breather by instinct, but this ability is quickly lost when he becomes subjected to his modern-day environment.

Yoga breathing is slow, deep and rhythmical; air is inhaled and exhaled through the nose, with mouth closed. This is an elementary rule of correct breathing. The nose is the guardian of the inner door, but the most important task of this organ is the absorption of prana from the air. You inhale air through the nasal channels; the mucus membranes with their secretions filter it of dust particles; and then it is carried by the bronchial tubes directly to the lungs. By this process the oxygen is not only filtered, but also warmed up by the time it reaches its destination. Then by exhalation through the nose again, the carbon dioxide, or waste material, is eliminated.

This fresh oxygen inhaled through the nostrils provides a supply for proper blood circulation. The blood, refreshed and purified by oxygen, moves on from the lungs to the heart via arteries, blood vessels, and capillaries, reaching every cell in the body. It stimulates the endocrine glands, it rebuilds tissues, it feeds the nerves, it helps to digest food. And then, having performed its duties of collecting impurities and waste materials, it travels back through the veins to the lungs. This process repeats itself every three minutes.

We seem to know the rules, and still we go on abusing this wonderful body of ours, and refuse to use it to its full capacity. Few people breathe properly, they don't inhale enough oxygen, and thus can't get rid of waste material, which results in poor health. Without sufficient oxygen the body functions are slowed down, and the tissues have a much more difficult task to renew themselves.

Maybe we should re-educate ourselves. I realize it is not an easy task, since we were taught so many bad habits which civilized man adopted without giving much thought to their consequences. For instance, consider our diet, the wrong foods with which we endulge ourselves with joy, our smoking habits, our excessive drinking of alcoholic beverages. We forget to exercise, have no time to take a walk, and even less time to swim or play games. Modern man is so busy with his financial gains and material possessions that he has forgotten his most precious possession . . . his body and his well being.

Man derives more energy from the air he breathes than from any other single source. What keeps the brain going, the heart pumping, the digestion working, the blood circulating? In short, what keeps a human being alive? Oxygen! Proper breathing could vastly increase the body's resistance to mental and physical complaints, giving the body new health and vitality. Life and breath are synonymous. I read somewhere that it was said by a Yogi: "Life enters by the nostrils, death by the mouth."

Yoga exercises are done with deep breathing; otherwise there is hardly any benefit experienced from them. A student of mine practiced yoga for about two years from books and a television program she watched from time to time. She paid little attention to proper breathing techniques, concentrating mainly on the postures. When she joined my class, her health was in poor shape and arthritis in her hands and joints was causing her much pain. Her bones cracked each time she tried to bend. She confessed taking seven to eight painkillers a day. Two years of yoga without the proper breathing and proper instructions had not been too helpful. After a few months of practicing Yoga with deep rhythmic breathing, and following a simple diet, the pain subsided and the cracking of the bones was reduced. In fact, she needed no painkillers any more.

There is another case worth mentioning. Mrs. J., who had high blood pressure, started to take lessons at age 59. She was stiff and clumsy, and negative on top of it. "I can never do these postures," she said. Of course, she soon learned most of the asanas quite well and her breathing became perfect. After a few months of working steadily at Yoga exercises, she had her doctor check her blood pressure and he found it normal. He and my student were pleased with the outcome. I could record many such cases I witnessed since I have been teaching Yoga.

It is very important to think positively while exercising and to believe in satisfactory results. Any doubts will detain the person from accomplishing the goal. When the student believes that Yoga will help to restore his or her poor health, it usually works.

What happens when we do take a deep rhythmic breath, inhaling through the nostrils and exhaling through the nostrils? According to the Yogis, who have watched the functioning of the body, a deep rhythmic breath exerts a mild pressure upon the liver, stomach, and digestive tract which acts like a mild massage, aiding the proper relation of the pressure in the organs and in the abdomen.

It is evident that the mere exercising of the surface muscles, as it is done in Western systems of physical culture, is not enough. The inner organs need to be exercised as well. When deep rhythmic breathing is done the Yoga way, the diaphragm becomes strengthened and assumes proper functioning.

Swimming and baseball as well as other sports are good for you, but your breathing during these activities is usually jerky and unsystematic. Thus the greater quantity of oxygen obtained by the lungs is dissipated immediately and one experiences loss of energy. For this reason, after participating in these various sports, a person gets tired and often short of breath.

The same can be said about professional players who seem to make good use of their muscles and joints and do plenty of running and exercising. Nevertheless, as they mature, in many cases they have to give up participating professionally because of poor health. Arthritis is common among these men, and colds are quite prevalent. If physical exertion alone would keep the body healthy, then they wouldn't have so many common illnesses.

The Yoga way of breathing refreshes you, as it has a revitalizing effect on glands and vital organs. It also has a calming effect on the nervous system and brain. This explains why after practicing Yoga exercises with deep breathing one feels rested and relaxed. It is remarkable how often a student arrives for a Yoga lesson looking tired and stiff, and after a few Yoga postures with deep breathing begins to look different. Even his face projects a peaceful expression.

The other day a business man, a student of mine, arrived at the studio looking very tired. "I wonder whether I'll be able to do anything today, I am so tired," he said. At the end of the class he exclaimed: "I'm ready to start all over again. I feel wonderful now." He is no exception. Most of my students feel this way.

In the March 1968 edition of *The Reader's Digest,* I read Dr. Kenneth H. Cooper's article, condensed from *Aerobics.* In it, Dr. Cooper said: "The best kind of 'fitness' is what we call endurance fitness: the ability to do prolonged work without fatigue. It has to do with the body's over-all health, the health of the heart, the lungs, the health of the entire cardiovascular system and the other organs, as well as the muscles. The key to the whole thing is *oxygen.*"

The Yogis, thousands of years ago, arrived at the opinion that the quality of the blood depends to a great extent on the quantity of oxygen absorbed by the lungs. Faulty breathing, therefore, has a direct influence upon the quality of the blood which, in turn, affects all the organs of the body. The stomach and digestive organs especially are affected by insufficient oxygen due to faulty breathing.

When we do shallow breathing we somehow use up more energy. This might explain why people are tired by the end of the day. It has been said by the Yogis that during sleeping hours we breathe deeply and rhythmically, without being aware of it. Upon arising, we don't remember this and return to shallow breathing unless we have studied the yoga way.

The Yogis have also adopted the conception that *nature* and *man* are indisputably functioning as *one!* Sun and Moon are considered to be part of the human body. The Sun flows through the right nostril, and the Moon flows through the left nostril. Try closing the right nostril and blowing through the left one, the Moon. Hold your palm in front of it—you will feel cool air blown out. The opposite will be experienced with the other nostril. The Sun will blow out much warmer air.

Definite changes begin to take place when you practice and study Yoga seriously. But it is necessary to discipline the emotions and follow a certain pattern to keep the body healthy and the mind peaceful. Qualities developed by means of yoga breathing, Yoga postures, relaxation, concentration, and meditation lead to serenity of spirit and mastery of *oneself.*

WHAT "RHYTHMIC BREATHING" MEANS

1. Rhythm is determined by your own pulsebeat. To establish your rhythm, take a count of your pulse aloud—one-two-three-four—repeating it a few times. At the start count only to four. Then begin to count mentally until you are absolutely sure that you have caught the rhythm of your pulse. When you begin the actual exercises, count mentally, but don't

keep your attention on it; it should become an unconscious habit.
2. Breathe through the nose by slightly contracting the throat (this will partially close the epiglottis), and keep your mouth closed. There should be a slight hissing sound in the back of the throat. Never raise your chest while inhaling. Your abdomen should be pushed out slightly. Your rib cage should expand on both sides. Now slowly exhale with the same hissing sound while contracting your rib cage and pulling in your stomach slightly.
3. Begin to count mentally four pulsebeats while inhaling, then hold for two pulsebeats, and exhale on four pulsebeats. Your breath should flow smoothly and rhythmically. Remember, "four-in-and-four-out" is one exercise. Repeat, in the beginning five times per session.
4. Eventually, you will increase the amount to sixty exercises a day, but never during one session. They should be divided into two or three sessions. We start moderately, increasing the amount of oxygen in the body until the system gets adjusted to this additional oxygen. At first, it might create a feeling of dizziness, which you might blame on yoga. Therefore, I want you to work slowly at it and derive as much benefit as possible from the breathing exercises.

The Complete Yoga Breathing

Inhale, activating the diaphragm, pushing the abdomen outward. The pushing-out movement will fill the lower part of the lungs with air. This will expand the lower ribs and the middle of the thorax, which gradually take over the air from the lower part of your lungs.

Begin the exhalation, drawing the abdomen in. This lifts the diaphragm, the rib cage returns to normal position, and the air is expelled from the lungs, carrying with it the carbon dioxide from your body.

Breathe in and out smoothly, not with a jerky movement. The exhalation is also done through the nose (mouth closed). Every part of the lungs is filled with air, increasing the intake of oxygen.

The rhythmic breathing exercises, which you are to practice, after you have mastered the Yoga breathing described above, with every posture, can be found starting on page 50.

BREATHING EXERCISES FOR BEGINNERS AND ADVANCED STUDENTS

The following exercises are practiced inhaling and exhaling through the nose, mouth closed, and in a standing position.

1. Breathing Exercise

a.   Inhale, rising up on the tips of your toes. Hold your breath while standing on your toes. Exhale while slowly lowering the heels to the floor (Figure 1–a).

b.   Inhale, rising on the tips of your toes. Hold your breath while standing; exhale while lowering the body to a squatting position (Figure 1–b). Stand up.

c.   Inhale, raising both arms above the head, palms together (Figure 1–c). Stretch. Hold your breath for a moment. While exhaling, drop your arms (Figure 1–cc).

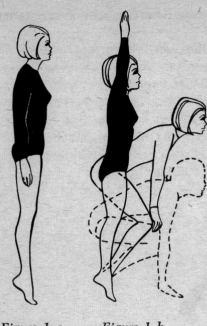

Figure 1-a   Figure 1-b

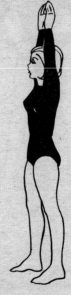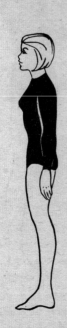

Figure 1-c   Figure 1-cc

d.   Inhale, bringing your palms together in front of your chest; hold your breath for a moment (Figure 1–d). Exhale, raising arms above your head, palms still together. Look up. Inhale again, and slowly bring arms back to starting position, exhaling as you do.

e.   Inhale, hands on hips. Exhale, bending forward (Figure 1–e). Return to upright position. Inhale, bend backwards as far as you can, then exhale. Return to upright position.

f.   Inhale, hands on hips. Exhale, and bend sideways (Figure 1–f), first to the right and then to the left.

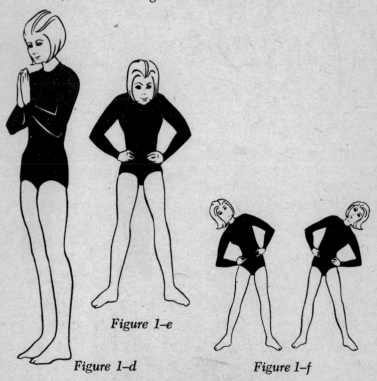

Figure 1–e

Figure 1–d

Figure 1–f

Each of these breathing exercises should be done from three to five times. Each return to starting position counts one. You can increase the number with experience.

2. Breathing Exercise

a) Sit on the floor tailor fashion or in the Lotus pose.
b) Spine straight.
c) Eyes closed.
d) Concentrate on your breathing, leaving all thoughts out and putting your mind at rest.
   Inhale slowly through the nose on count of four, hold on count of two, and then slowly exhale through the nose on count of four again.
f) Repeat three times.
g) With each inhalation visualize the marvellous prana, or life energy, entering your body, bringing health, beauty, and peace into your whole being.
h) And with each exhalation, visualize all the waste material, the carbon dioxide, leaving your body through all the pores, your fingers and toes.

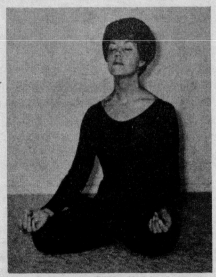

Phyllis Samson, student and assistant

3. *Breathing Exercise Using the Blowing Method*

a)   Remain in the same position as in the No. 2 exercise.
b)   Take a deep breath.
c)   Hold it for a while—as long as you feel comfortable without strain on the chest.
d)   Then start breathing out, using a different method—first blow up your cheeks, and then start blowing through pursed lips.

Repeat two or three times. It strengthens the muscles of the diaphragm.

4. *Breathing Exercise Using the Whistle*

a)   Sit in the position as in postures 2 and 3.
b)   Inhale deeply.
c)   Hold your breath as long as possible.
d)   Then start exhaling in the following manner: purse your lips and kind of whistle out the breath. It is a cleansing way of breathing and good for the nervous system.

5. *Cleansing Breathing Exercises*

The following breathing exercises are done while standing, legs apart, inhaling rhythmically through the nose, but exhaling through the mouth in rhythmical staccato, forming forcefully a sound of "ha-ha-ha-ha!" (This is known as a "cleansing breath" because it cleanses the respiratory organs.)

a.   Inhale, stretch both arms out in front, then swing them back and up (Figure 2–a). Exhale through the mouth, drop the arms.

b.   Inhale, stretch your arms forward, palms down. Holding your breath, move arms sideways, lifting the shoulders slightly, and then forward again several times (Figure 2–b). Drop the arms, exhaling with the mouth open. Exercises (a) and (b) are of great help in controlling nervous trembling of the hands or head.

c.   Inhale, place your fingertips on your shoulders and, while holding your breath, join your elbows on your chest, then move them wide apart several times (Figure 2–c). Exhale through the mouth.

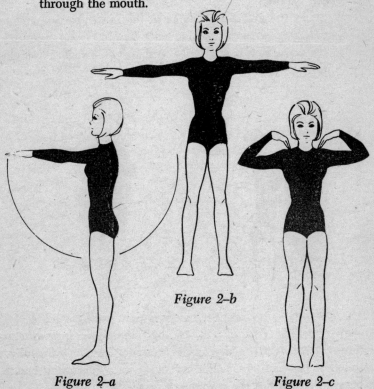

Figure 2–b

Figure 2–a

Figure 2–c

d. Inhale, stretch your arms forward, hold your breath, and begin to swing your arms like a windmill a few times in one direction (Figure 2–d). Exhale through the open mouth. Repeat, swinging in the opposite direction.

e. Inhale, move your arms backwards until your hands meet. Clench your fists (Figure 2–e). Hold your breath and bend forward, stretching arms behind. Exhale through the nose and return to starting position.

f. Stand straight. Clasp your fingers around the neck. Inhale deeply. Holding your breath, start twisting twice to the right, and then twice to the left. The lower part of the body doesn't move. Then exhale forcefully through the mouth.

g. Stand straight. Keep fingers in the same position. Inhale deeply. And now, holding your breath, swing sideways, twice to the left and twice to the right. Exhale forcefully through the mouth.

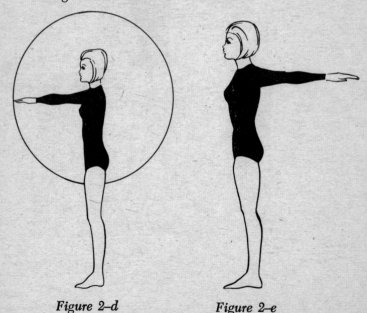

Figure 2–d   Figure 2–e

h.   Stand straight. Inhale deeply and stretch both arms in front of you, palms away from your body (Figure 2–h). Holding your breath, keep stretching one hand at a time forward, from the shoulder. Exhale forcefully through the mouth. Repeat a few times and relax. A good way to relax after these exercises is to let your head fall forward and keep it in this position for a few moments.

Each of these exercises should be done three to five times. Each return to starting position counts one. Again, you can increase the number with experience.

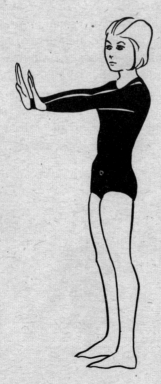

Figure 2–h

ALTERNATE BREATHING EXERCISES—
ANULOMA VILOMA PRANAYAMA

6. Single Nostril Breathing

Sit with a straight spine in tailor fashion or in a Lotus pose, completely relaxed with closed eyes. Close the right nostril with the thumb of the right hand. Inhale through the left nostril to the count of five. Do this without making any noise. Without holding the breath, exhale through the same nostril twice as many times; if you inhaled to the count of five, exhale ten counts —counting mentally, of course. Repeat six times at first and increase the number as time goes on. Alternate, using the same method with the left nostril, but hold the left nostril with the last two fingers of the right hand. The number of rounds can be increased, and also the number of intakes of breath can be increased. For instance, inhale six and exhale twelve, and then inhale eight and exhale sixteen. The idea is always to exhale a double amount.

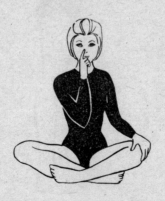

7. Both Nostrils Breathing

After you have practiced the single nostril alternate breathing for several weeks, try a different method. However, remember that in order to do this breathing exercise you must be relaxed and your mind at rest and peace. Also you cannot allow your thoughts to wander from object to object. You must keep your thoughts concentrated on the prana you are inhaling into your body. It is done as follows: Sitting in the same position as before, close the right nostril with the right thumb. Inhale through the left nostril, and then immediately close the left nostril with your right ring finger and little finger. Then remove your thumb and exhale through the right nostril.

Repeat immediately, inhaling through the right nostril while holding the left, and then exhaling through the left.

Always use double counts for exhalation, just as in the single nostril breathing exercise. And go very slowly before you increase the amount of inhalation. This is an excellent method of breathing, but it should be done in the presence of an experienced teacher, who understands what impact it has on the brain and the mind. I would not suggest that anyone attempt to do it alone.

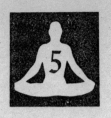

Recapture Youth
with Yoga

The practice of the *asanas* will help to attain perfection, concentration of mind and unfold various psychic powers. Men, women and children regardless of age can study some form of yoga, since the exercises refresh the body rather than tire it. The idea is to stimulate the functions of glands, nerves, the main muscles of the body, including the heart, without fatiguing them. This ancient science brings health to brain and body.

The fundamental difference between yoga exercises and ordinary exercises is that the latter emphasize violent movements of muscles, whereas in the yoga system all movements are slow and gradual with proper breathing and relaxation, thus age doesn't enter into consideration. One can start as young as five and as old as 80.

Since the main purpose of exercise is to increase the circulation and the intake of oxygen, in Hatha Yoga this is achieved through the simple movements of the spine and various joints of the body, with deep rhythmic breathing, systematic stretching, tensing and relaxing of all the muscles of the body.

Yoga exercises combined with the deep rhythmic breathing are designed to draw blood to the spine, with the result that the nerves which emanate from the spine are toned up. The forward and backward bending postures and the lateral ones not only send up blood to the brain, but also stimulate the many other organs of the body. Thus people who suffer from arthritis of the spine have been greatly helped by the rhythmic bends and twistings that increase the mobility of the limbs. Pressures on nerves, caused by subtle misalignment and vertebral maladjustments are often relieved.

Feel tired or tense or restless? Yoga will help you to overcome these emotional disturbances and find peace of mind by learning the methods of relaxation. By practicing yoga daily you can control your weight problems, whether overweight or underweight.

Self-discipline is one of the many merits you can obtain by being a devoted yoga student.

A better posture and a slender figure make you look younger and have a happier attitude. As you read in the previous chapter, Hatha-Yoga training consists of correct deep rhythmic breathing, asanas, for bodily coordination, exercises for mental and physical relaxation, concentration, meditation and proper diet.

The Yogis say that no one is completely healthy unless his heart, lungs, brain, liver, kidneys, eyes and hearing are functioning perfectly. A person with strong muscles is not necessarily a healthy specimen. The internal organs actually determine the health of an individual. A person with highly developed muscles can still be weak and ill from a serious disease.

Thus, the Yogis evolved certain postures which, when coupled with deep rhythmic breathing exercises, keep the nervous system working efficiently. These postures practiced daily bring positive benefits. According to Yogis, a body suffering aches and pains cannot enjoy a full life or even concentrate in peace. A body must be fit and in perfect health to be ready for spiritual progress.

The exercises originally designed by the old masters were based on observing the motions of animals. They became aware that animals have the capacity to relax completely and remain motionless with perfect ease. Thus, many of the postures became known as Camel, Lion, Cobra, Peacock, Crocodile, Fish, Cat, Locust exercise and so on.

Each posture was created for a definite part of the body, to stimulate the workings of an individual organ during the exercises. This in turn was supposed to promote a supply of additional blood to these organs while doing the particular posture. The theory and practice of yoga rose out of practical necessity answering the need of man. Man is irresistibly drawn toward the ideal of perfection.

Yoga exercises bring results without strenuous physical activity.

Nevertheless, anyone with a chronic disease who has never exercised before should definitely ask first for medical advice.

Yoga exercises will help tone the muscles and keep the body firm. Firmness of the muscles is determined by the time devoted to exercising. The less we work at it, the flabbier muscles become. Sometimes flabby muscles appear to be fat and one looks out of proportion. By returning the muscles to their normal condition these added inches in measurement disappear. A fat person appears years older than his actual age.

Appearance these days is vital, because people are so conscious of age. Age determines many aspects of life—your job, your marriage, your sexual life. Janet Blair, a movie star, in an interview with Lydia Lane of the *Los Angeles Times* of July 30, 1967, said: "If you don't exercise, you spread. I am disciplined about working out seven days a week. Not long—10 or 15 minutes—but I am consistent, and this is what counts."

There are easy postures for the beginners, more complicated ones to follow later on. The form does not determine its results, but the repetition of the daily routine. Exercises must be done regularly. And a good point of yoga is that no gadgets are required. All you need are a mat and comfortable slacks or leotards. As Dr. Paul Dudley White has said: "It matters little, if at all, what type of exercise it is, provided it suits the strength and liking of the individual concerned. It is well to establish a regular habit and to maintain it through thick and thin. One should regard it just as essential to good health as eating, sleeping, and working."

Thousands of yoga students all over the world are gaining tremendous benefits from these techniques. The postures are simple and logical, and anyone with a sound body can accomplish them. Some of the postures are much easier than many Western forms of exercises.

Gloria Swanson has said that her health and beauty secret is yoga. Yehudi Menuhin considered yoga to be as important to his art as his violin practice. Mrs. Wyatt Cooper, another enormously attractive stander-on-head, says: "I can do it for four or five minutes."

I read in Vogue's issue of April 15th, 1967, about an international beauty known for her indefatigable chic along with a thousand other talents who was willing to disclose an energy secret, a "simple yoga exercise." She suggested: "Sit on the floor cross-legged, back straight, body relaxed and do your breathing exercises."

Perfectly reasonable men and women today are engaged in practicing yoga exercises. We find lawyers, business men and women, bankers and even doctors among the enthusiastic students. Of course, the well-known beauties such as Marion Mill Preminger (Mrs. Mayer), Dolores Del Rio, Greto Garbo, Olivia de Havilland, Jennifer Jones and, as I already mentioned before, Gloria Swanson have been using yoga for a long time to good effect. Many famous male stars also have been practicing yoga lately.

The new Prime Minister of Canada, Mr. Trudeau, practices yoga. Before his election in an interview he spoke about it, saying yoga definitely helps the mind and body jointly to cope with emergencies.

My students in all walks of life respond well. Only recently I met a seventeen-year-old youngster. At the age of fifteen he was expelled from school, because he was constantly getting into fights with other youngsters. In one fight his nose was broken. Being expelled affected his nervous system, and his blood pressure went up to 200. His parents tried every means to help this boy. The broken nose was never set correctly as he was afraid to have it done.

After two months of yoga, his thinking has changed. The blood pressure returned to normal and he has even had his nose corrected, too. I am sure that the principal of the school will reconsider his case and accept him back, for the boy is now eager to finish his high school education. In the meantime he has won a trophy as the best accordian player in California.

Yoga teaches discipline and control of emotions. This takes us to the next step of detachment from fear, anxiety and worries that make life difficult and unpleasant. Of course, to accomplish anything one has to have the strong need for it, and work at it. Nothing comes easy in life. Perseverance, faith, determination and a little bit of encouragement will do it.

Another student of mine, a married lady and mother of two children suddenly got tired of her husband. No matter what he tried to do, she saw it in a negative light. She even suspected him of having a love affair with another woman and she was ready to jump into the divorce court. She started to take yoga lessons. Her face was always pensive and she had a hard time in relaxing. But as she continued and gained confidence to was in her behavior, not in her husband's. It is so easy to blame confide in me, I was able to make her understand the fault that others, but not so simple to admit our own shortcomings. Today she and her husband are very happy and the whole family is doing yoga now.

Oxygen is the most vital food for fueling the body and mind for everyday function. Proper exercise through coordination of various joints, relaxation, discipline of mind, natural foods and a simple diet are the basis of yoga training. But it must be remembered that the exercises and the deep rhythmic breathing should be practiced together in order that the additional supply of oxygen thus brought into our system will cause our glands, muscles and nerves to function better.

The laws of health are the laws of Nature on which yoga is based. The yogi teachers of India insisted that unless the body is fit the mind cannot function to its fullest capacity. Patanjali, considered the father of yoga, was the first to write down in Sanskrit language what was told from teacher to student year after year: "Yoga gives us power to control mental waves such as sadness, depression, anger and unrest. These waves arise from any kind of mental disturbance. The person who learns to control these waves has conquered life itself."

The science of yoga prevails over forces that obstruct one's goal. In other words, systematic training in yoga will lead you to understand *how to live a longer life,* how to gain control over your body and undesirable habits. The person who works at it steadily with faith and conviction arrives eventually at a state of consciousness that transcends the limits of the flesh.

Yoga is basically a "way of life" which enables one to conserve energy and coordinate the power of body, power of mind, power of soul. Rejuvenation through yoga will be your guide to a more rewarding life. You will attain physical and mental youthfulness, and discover a new and thrilling feeling of your inner self, which might be asleep within you. A chance of second youth with an added vitality will clear up many obstacles, and you will find serenity and peace of mind. Calendar age shouldn't bother you. There is no reason why all the benefits from this ancient wisdom should not be yours. The new life you might be in search of can be yours, as you have the power to recondition your body and reconstruct your thoughts.

We all search for the proverbial fountain of youth at some time in our lives. The Hunza people have proven that longevity could be a normal experience, even in our society. Who would resist the possibility of living a longer and healthier life?

A FEW BASIC RULES TO FOLLOW

1. Wear comfortable clothes.
2. Exercise in a well-ventilated room, or outdoors if the weather permits.
3. Choose a surface that is not too hard or too soft. Use a blanket or a mat to exercise on.

4. Exercises should be done on an empty stomach, the first thing upon arising or before retiring.

5. The postures are done lying, sitting or standing. However, they also can be done sitting in a chair, if one has difficulties in getting to the floor, at least in the beginning until the muscles are more at rest.

6. Exercises also can be done lying on a couch or a bed. A slant board is useful for those having trouble getting to the floor. (A slant board is good for anyone, as the principle is to keep the head down.) It is very relaxing.

7. Until you reach perfection, practice only a few postures at one time; do the ones that are easy for you. Then, after you have made progress, include the others.

8. Fifteen to thirty minutes are sufficient for an average session. If you don't have that much time, even five minutes a day will prove beneficial. But never miss a day.

9. Do not exercise more than a total of one hour a day.

10. Rest in between the various postures so that you don't get tired. These postures are designed to give you a feeling of comfort and relaxation, not fatigue. Every posture should be combined with deep rhythmic breathing.

11. Relax the body before you begin to exercise.

12. Rest and sleep are of paramount importance for the program to work effectively. Sleep before midnight is considered the best.

13. If you have any health problems, be sure to consult your doctor before you begin to exercise.

14. Good food and a sensible diet are quite essential, too.

FIRST WEEK
EXERCISES OR ASANAS (IN SANSKRIT)

The Bridge—Sethu Bandhasana

I. a. Lie flat on your back. Pull up feet along the floor as close to the body as possible, knees and heels together.

  b. Inhale slowly and raise the body as high as you can (Figure 1–1).

  c. Hold the breath and remain in this position for two to four seconds.

  d. Exhale slowly, lowering the body to the floor. Repeat three times and eventually increase to ten.

II. a. After you have practiced (Figure 1–1) for a while and feel comfortable in this position, you can try a more advanced pose.

  b. Build a longer bridge by stretching your feet further out (Figure 1–2).

  c. Inhale, raising the body (Figure 3), hold briefly, then exhale and return to starting position. Repeat at least five times.

This posture strengthens the back. It is beneficial to anyone who suffers from sacroiliac pain, tired or aching back. In time it will increase the circulation. Whenever you feel a discomfort in the back region, practice the bridge. But remember never to strain any part of the body or muscle. It should be done with ease, gracefully and always accompanied by deep rhythmic breathing.

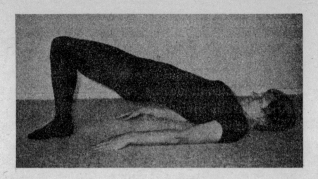

Figure 1–1

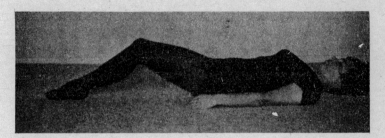

Figure 1–2

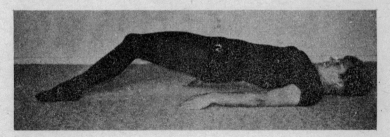

Figure 1–3

Marsha Carr, a student

Wind Relieving Posture—*Vatayanasana*

I. a. Lie flat on the floor (Figure 2–1).
   b. Inhale, draw in the right knee and pull it onto your chest with both hands (Figure 2–2).
   c. Hold your breath for two seconds while stretching the leg up (Figure 2–3).
   d. Exhale and slowly return to starting position.
   e. Alternate and do the same with the left leg. Repeat twice with each leg.

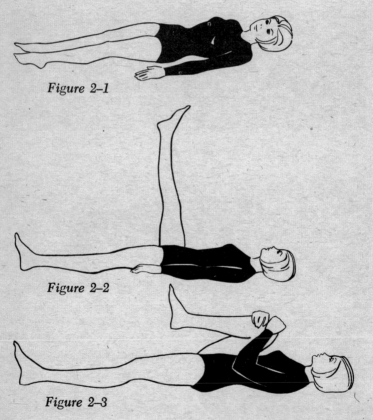

Figure 2–1

Figure 2–2

Figure 2–3

II. Variation:
   a. Inhale, draw both knees in (Figure 2–4).
   b. Hold your breath while stretching both legs up (Figure 2–5).
   c. Exhale and slowly return to starting position. Repeat twice.

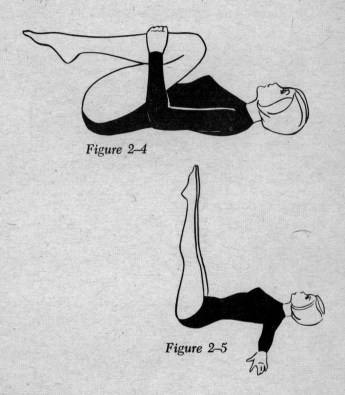

Figure 2–4

Figure 2–5

In the beginning don't try to do more than twice, as the principle muscles at work are the upper and lower abdominals. The muscles should be strengthened gradually to avoid any discomfort. This posture is also beneficial to relieve gas pain, regulate constipation troubles and, above all, help to strengthen abdominal muscles, giving the figure a thinner and younger look.

The Reverse Posture—Viparita Karani Mudra

a.   Lie flat on your back (Figure 3–1).
b.   Start slowly raising legs, supporting the body with both hands (Figure 3–2).
c.   Continue to raise legs (Figure 3–3).

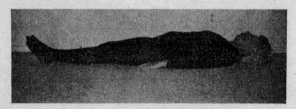

Figure 3–1   Jessie Agena

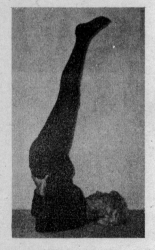

Figure 3–2

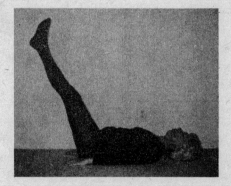

Figure 3–3

d. Eyes closed, the deep breathing should be done slowly through the nose, inhaling and exhaling rhythmically. Hold the position for at least one minute. Eventually it should be increased to 5 minutes.

e. Then, slowly start coming down, bending the knees first (Figure 3–4). Relax.

f. In case you have difficulties in raising the body at start, a wall can be used, or a piece of furniture heavy enough to support the body. Feet in this position, lean against the edge of the object (Figure 3–5). The next step is to raise the body with both arms.

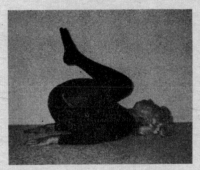

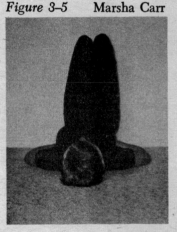

Figure 3–5   Marsha Carr

Figure 3–4   Jessie Agena

This posture has a rejuvenating effect on the facial muscles and a beautifying effect on the skin. It brings the blood to the upper part of the body, stimulating the thyroid glands. It also stimulates the gonad or sex glands. This exercise is vital to both men and women.

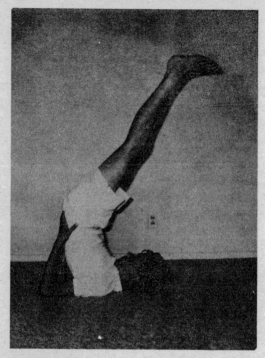

Figure 3–6 Chris Dunn

Lotus Pose—Padmasana

This posture is the symbol of yoga (Figure 4–1) and used during meditation. It has a calming effect on the mind. It is done as follows:

a. Sit on the floor, both legs extended.

b. Pick up the right foot with both hands and place it on the left thigh (Figure 4–2).

c. When the right knee is flat on the floor, at this point, then you can try to bring the left foot to the right thigh, by bending the knee first.

d. Keep spine erect, hands over the knees with palms open, thumb and forefinger rounded. However, at night, reverse the position of the palms, holding them down.

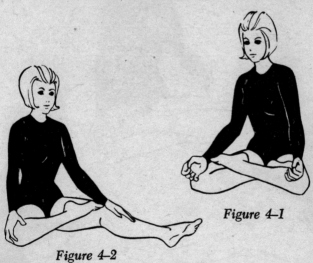

Figure 4–1

Figure 4–2

This is the complete Lotus pose. It should *never* be tried by force. At first try to sit a few seconds only, until you feel comfortable in it.

Until you can assume the Lotus pose properly, sit tailor fashion (Figure 4–3). The difference of this pose is the position of the heels. In Sanskrit it is called the Siddhasana.

To practice the Lotus pose, first you should work on the Half-Lotus pose (Figure 4–4).

a. The right foot is placed on the left thigh.
b. Bounce the knee up and down, helping to push it down closer to the floor with the hand. It should be done daily. The joints will eventually become flexible.
c. Reverse the pose (Figure 4–5).

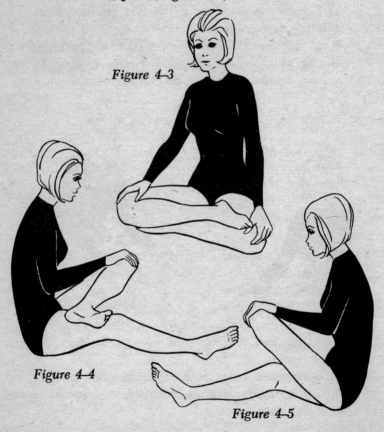

Figure 4–3

Figure 4–4

Figure 4–5

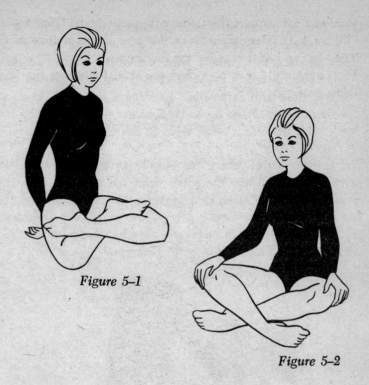

Figure 5–1

Figure 5–2

The Stoop or Yoga Mudra

I. a. Sit tailor fashion or Lotus pose. Spine straight. Hands clasped behind the back (Figure 5–1 or 5–2).
   b. Inhale slowly and rhythmically. Eyes closed. Concentrate on the benefits you are deriving from the prana.
   c. Then hold the breath briefly and start exhaling, bending forwards until your forehead touches the floor (Figure 5–3).
   d. In the beginning do this slowly, without force.
   e. Return to starting position, also very slowly, and repeat this pose three times.

II. a. Remain in the same position sitting straight with hands clasped in the back.

b. Inhale as in the above pose, and when you start exhaling bend forward to the right knee, trying to bring your face as close to it as possible, touching it with your forehead or the tip of the nose. Then repeat the same to the left knee. Practice it a few times to develop flexibility.

The benefits derived from this posture are many. It tones the pelvic region. It keeps the colon clean and many find a relief from constipation. Thus, it is important to concentrate on the parts of the body involved in this posture, mainly the abdominal region and the colon. In fact, every exercise should be practiced with deep concentration to get the best results.

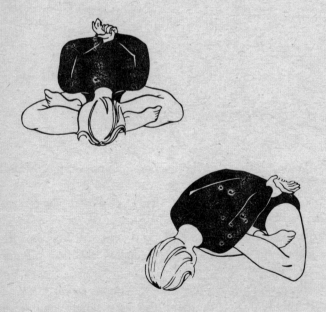

Figure 5–3

Legs and Arms Stretching Exercises—Hastha Padasan

a. Sit straight, legs stretched and apart, arms above the head (Figure 6–1).
b. Inhale deeply and hold the breath for a few seconds.
c. Exhale, slowly bending down, trying to catch the toes, or the sole of your foot (Figure 6–2).

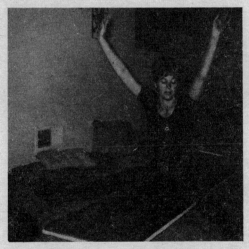

Figure 6–1   Marsha Carr

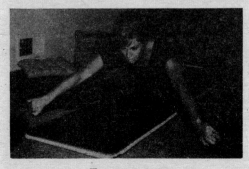

Figure 6–2

d. Beginners, until your head rests on the floor, should rock the back to get more flexibility.

e. Return to starting position.

f. Remain in the same position with hands stretched above the head and this time bend to the right knee until the tip of your nose touches it, hands holding on to the ankle (Figure 6–3).

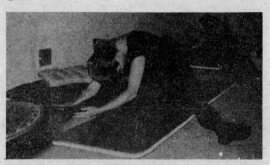

Figure 6–3

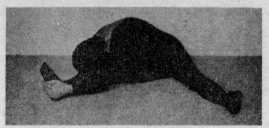

Figure 6–4 Phyllis Sampson

g. Advanced students follow (Figure 6–4), clasping hands around the foot.

h. Now, repeat the same bending to the left knee. Each time the same breathing technique should be used and practiced patiently until flexibility has been accomplished.

Benefits derived from this asana are numerous. It helps to keep the spine stretched, also the vertebrae of the entire spinal cord.

It strengthens the muscles of the shoulders, upper back and arms. It is weight reducing, as the stomach muscles are involved in these various positions. It brings circulation into the sacroiliac, relieving it from pressure. While you inhale, visualize the wonderful health prana is bringing into the body, and then as you exhale, visualize the waste material leaving the body.

Neck Exercises

I. a. Sit tailor fashion or in the Lotus pose on the floor, spine straight and relaxed, the shoulders not moving.
   b. Throw your head forward (Figure 7–1).
   c. Then throw the head backwards (Figure 7–2). Repeat this at least ten times.

II. a. Turn the head to the right with a slight jerk, then straight; now turn the head to the left, and straight. Here again work the neck only—shoulders don't move. Repeat five times.

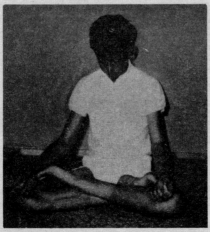

Figure 7–1   Chris Dunn

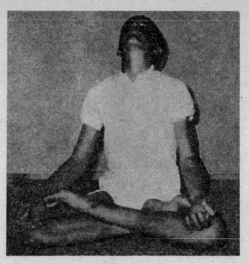

Figure 7-2

III. a. Tilt the head sideways to the right, ear to shoulder, then straight. Repeat the same to the left side and straight. Repeat at least five times.

IV. a. Rotate your head clockwise a few times and then reverse doing it counterclockwise a few times. It should be done slowly with a complete feeling of relaxation.

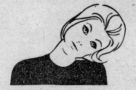 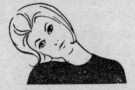

These simple movements release tension around the neck and are very effective. You can practice them at any time during the day, while you are taking a bath or sitting at your desk during office hours, or watching television. If you feel a noise in the back of your neck, sort of a gravel sound, while rotating your head, be sure to do these exercises daily, as it usually signifies that some unwanted deposits in the neck are slowing down your circulation. These movements will help you to correct this condition.

Another suggestion: these exercises can also be done with deep breathing. Then the technique is as follows: Inhale, moving into one direction and exhale, moving into the opposite direction. This can apply to all the above movements of the neck.

Eye Exercises

a. Remain in the same position as for the neck exercises.
b. Move your eyes up and then down slowly. Blink first, and then close eyes lightly. The face and head don't move.
c. Look to the right and then to the left. Blink and close eyes lightly. Here again, head doesn't move.
d. The corner of the right eye looks up, and then the corner of the left eye looks down. Blink and close the eyes lightly. Alternate the position.
e. Change vision by choosing an object close to the eyes, and then shift them to an object in the far distance. Blink and close the eyes lightly. Repeat each of these movements from six to ten times.

Remember to sit absolutely straight and relaxed. In each movement try to find a spot with your eyes and return to the same spot without moving the head or face. You can also do it as follows: After b, take a deep breath before you go on to the next movement. Follow each one with a deep breath. These exercises are quite helpful in improving your eyesight as they help to relax the eyes, and can be done any time your eyes feel tired.

Palming

a. Remain in the same position as for the eye exercises.
b. Place elbows on raised knees.
c. Close eyes lightly.
d. Spine straight.
e. Cover eyes with cupped hands.
f. Rest the heels of your palms on the cheekbones without pressing them, fingers crossed over the forehead.
g. Try to see black.

While in this position deep rhythmic breathing is suggested. Palm for about two to three minutes at a time. It relieves eye strain and is helpful for people who do a great deal of reading or figure work.

Arms, Hands and Fingers Exercises

a. Stand erect, relaxed, both hands at your sides.
b. Start shaking both hands simultaneously. Do it a few times.
c. Then turn both wrists clockwise, five times, and then turn them counterclockwise, the same number of times.
d. Then move each finger slowly, as though you are playing the piano. Repeat a few times.
e. Close your fists and tense them. Hold for a while, and then relax them. Repeat about five times.
f. Stretch both arms sideways, then bend the elbows, and stretch again. When you do stretch arms out, imagine that there is something in your way and you are trying to

push it away. It is effective and you will feel that stretch much more.

g. Repeat the same, stretching arms above your head toward the ceiling as if you are trying to move it, and then also in front of you.

Each exercise should be repeated a few times. By consciously tensing our hands and then letting go, we learn how to relax them and also the whole body. To be able to relax your hands when you are under pressure will somehow give you a feeling of relief. As we relax, after an experience of tension, the mind assumes that everything is all right and projects to the rest of the body a feeling of security. In fact, it is much easier to relieve tension through relaxation of muscles of the body, than trying to do it mentally.

Legs and Feet Exercises

a.   Stand erect. Both hands on the hips (Figure 11–1).

b.   Shake each foot, one at a time.

c.   Then turn the left ankle clockwise. After a few turns reverse it counterclockwise.

d.   Then same should be done with right ankle, following the same method.

e.   Stretch the right leg forward and then backward (Figure 11–2).

f.   Then stretch the right leg sideways (Figure 11–3). Repeat the same with left leg. Each position should be done five to ten times.

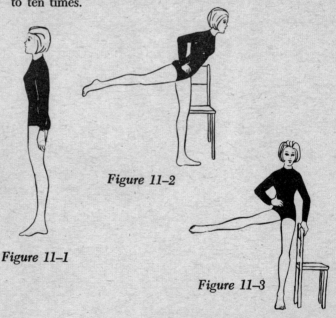

Figure 11–2

Figure 11–1

Figure 11–3

If necessary, to keep balance you can hold on to something sturdy. These exercises are excellent to keep legs and thighs in good shape. It also brings circulation into the feet and calves.

Head to Knee Exercises—*Padahasthasana*

I. a. Stand straight. Inhale and stretch arms above the head (Figure 12–1). Hold breath for a few seconds.

b. Exhale and start bending slowly forward, knees straight, hands grasping the toes, face pressing toward the knees (Figure 12–2). It should be done without any strain on the upper part of the body.

c. Inhale while you return to standing position and repeat three times.

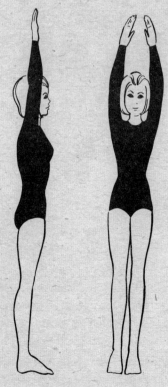

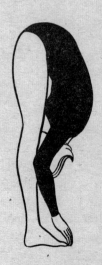

Figure 12–1   Figure 12–2

II.   Variation

With hands clasped in the back, feet apart, *inhale,* and bend down toward the left knee (Figure 12–3). Exhale while you are doing it. And then change toward the right knee. Repeat at least three times in each direction.

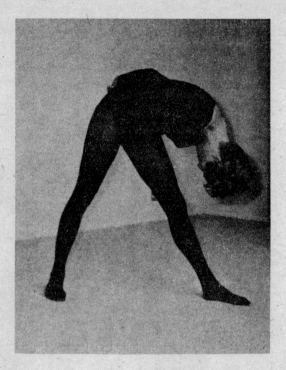

Figure 12–3

Anyone with a weak back or troubled disk should do exercise slowly and gradually until the back muscles get stronger and more flexible. These bending and stretching postures are excellent for the spine.

SECOND WEEK

Rocking Exercise

I. a. Sit on the floor. Draw in your legs, back round, head bent.
   b. Clasp hands under the knees (Figure 13–1).
   c. Rock forward and backwards. First start rocking backwards (Figures 13–2 and 13–3). Then rock forward.

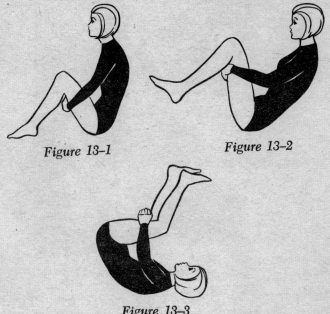

Figure 13–1   Figure 13–2

Figure 13–3

This posture is good for the spinal cord. It also helps to limber up the whole body. The spine should not be straight while rocking, otherwise it will be so much more difficult to get forward.

II. Variation

The advanced students should practice in the following manner:

a. Sit with legs criss-crossed. Hands clasp the opposite toes— left hand holds on to the right toes, right hand holds on to the left toes.

b. Now start rocking, first leaning forward trying to reach the floor with the face (Figure 13–4); then starting rocking backwards bringing feet over the head to the floor (Figure 13–5).

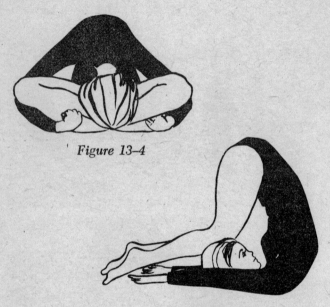

Figure 13–4

Figure 13–5

This posture looks difficult, but in reality it is not. It just requires some practice, and as one limbers up, it is done with ease. This posture gives a feeling of rhythm to your whole being. It also massages the vertebral column and stimulates the blood. It can also be done with deep breathing. Inhale, bending forward, and exhale, rolling backwards.

Crocodile Exercises

I. a. Lie flat on the floor, arms outstretched.
   b. Draw feet close to the body, knees bent (Figure 14–1).
   c. Inhale, turn the knees to the right and the face to the left, keeping the body flat on the floor (Figure 14–2).
   d. Exhale and reverse the posture: knees to the left and face to the right.
   e. Repeat 5 times.

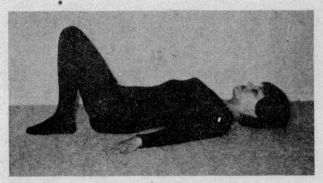

Figure 14–1   Phyllis Sampson

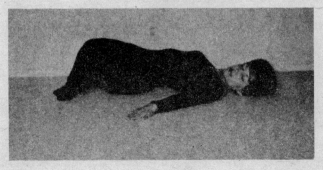

Figure 14–2

II. a. Still flat on the floor with arms stretched, criss-cross feet tightly.
   b. Inhale, twisting the lower part of the body to the right. Face and shoulders remain flat on the floor (Figure 14-3).
   c. Hold your breath for a few seconds.
   d. Exhale and reverse the position. Repeat three times. Relax.

III. a. Lie flat on the floor, hands outstretched, face and shoulders not moving. Place left foot on the right thigh (Figure 14-4).
   b. Inhale, turning the lower part of the body from the hips to the right (Figure 14-5). Hold the breath for three seconds.
   c. Exhale and reverse to the left side. Attempt to touch the floor in both instances, but don't force it. This is true concerning all three positions. Repeat 3 times.

These postures are good for the spine, the hips, legs and thighs. As the spine moves from side to side, it stretches all the muscles and stimulates the blood circulation. Eyes should be kept closed and the mind concentrated on the health and beauty your body is deriving from the exercises.

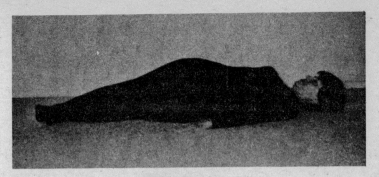

Figure 14-3

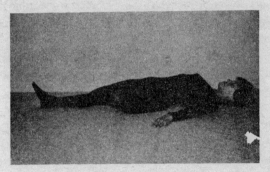

Figure 14-4

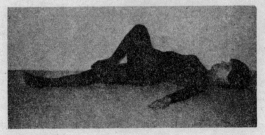

Figure 14-5

Head-Knee Pose—Janu Sirasana

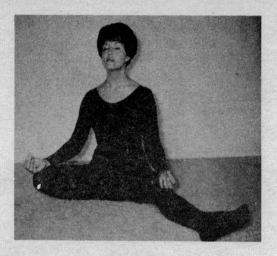

Figure 15–1

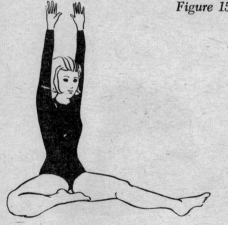

Figure 15–2

a.   Stretch both legs out and apart. Bend the left knee, bringing the left foot to the right thigh (Figure 15–1). Sit straight and relaxed.

b.   Inhale and stretch arms above the head (Figure 15–2).
c.   Then exhale and bend forward to the right knee. Catch
      toes of extended foot (Figure 15–3). Hold for five seconds
      or longer before you return to starting position.
d.   Reverse the posture and repeat the same with the other
      leg (Figure 15–4). Repeat three to six times on each side.

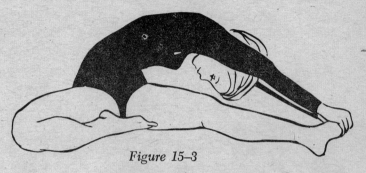

Figure 15–3

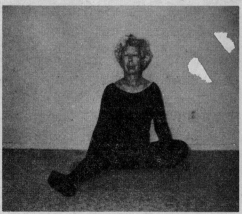

Figure 15–4   Jessie Agena

This exercise will help to limber up, to stretch your legs and
the muscles of the thighs. Beginners should not force when
bending down. Advanced students will be able to touch the knee
with the forehead shown in (Figure 15–3).

Cow Head Pose—Gomukhasana

a. Sit on the heels, knees together.
b. Raise the left arm and bend it behind your shoulders.
c. Now bend the right arm behind the back from the bottom and join the fingers together (Figure 16–1).
d. Inhale, sitting in this position.
e. Then exhale, bending forward (Figure 16–2). Hold the position for five to ten seconds, and then return to sitting on your heels.
f. Unlock the hands, and reverse the position. Repeat twice with each hand.

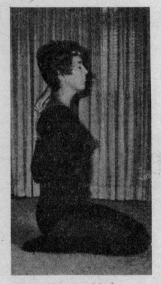

Figure 16–1

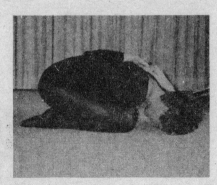

Figure 16–2

This asana is very good for people who have discomfort in the shoulder joints, as it might help to dissolve the calcium deposits, in case of bursitis. But practice without pulling too hard.

Good Posture Exercise

a. Sit on your heels, spine straight.
b. Bring both hands to the back.
c. Palms meet in the middle of the spine, fingers interlocked.
d. Inhale, stretching hands as far as you can away from the spine (Figure 17–1).
e. Now exhale, bending forward, continuing to stretch hands away from the body (Figure 17–2).
f. Relax in this position for five to ten seconds. Repeat twice.

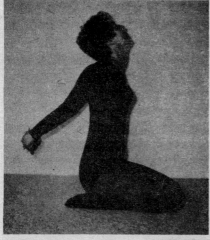

Figure 17–1   Ann Dunn

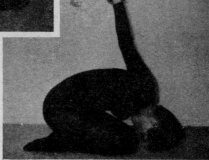

Figure 17–2

Star Posture

a.   Squat down.

b.   Cross left leg over the right leg and lay the right heel under the left thigh, while the left heel makes contact with the right thigh.

c.   Fold arms behind the back.

d.   Inhale, sitting in this position.

e.   Then exhale, bending forward (Figure 18–1).

f.   Hold this position for five to ten seconds. Return to starting position and repeat once more.

g.   Reverse the position of the legs and repeat the same.

This posture stimulates the nervous energy along the spine. It is also a beautifying position, as the blood rushes toward the face and head and feeds the facial tissues. Helpful to keep wrinkles away.

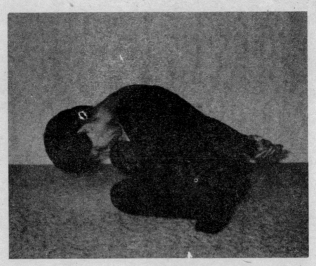

Figure 18–1   Phyllis Sampson

Shoulder-Stretching Posture

a. Sit tailor fashion, spine erect.

b. Stretch arms in front of you (Figure 19–1).

c. Inhale, clenching your fists and bringing them into the shoulders (Figure 19–2).

d. Hold your breath, bringing elbows together, in-and-out, three times.

e. Exhale, slowly bringing arms to starting position. Repeat again.

f. Relax, dropping your head slightly forward, and hold for a few seconds.

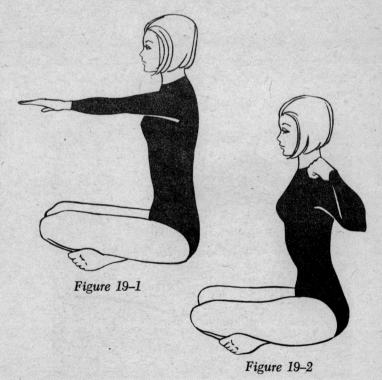

Figure 19–1

Figure 19–2

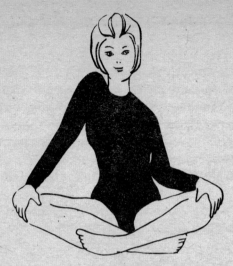

Figure 20-1

Shoulder Posture

a.   Sit tailor fashion, hands on knees.

b.   Inhale, raising the left shoulder as high as you comfortably can (Figure 20-1).

c.   Exhale, bringing the shoulder back to starting position. Repeat the same with right shoulder.

d.   Do the same with both shoulders. Repeat each twice.

This posture is excellent for the throat and neck vertebrae and for the shoulder blades.

Stomach Lift—Uddiyana Bandha and Nauli

a. Stand erect with the feet apart. Inhale deeply, then exhale completely. Pull in the abdomen so that it becomes hollow. Hold your breath. Bend the knees slightly and fall forward, hands on thighs (Figure 21–1).
b. Now pull the stomach in and out as long as you can hold the breath comfortably without breathing. Do not strain yourself. This can be repeated five times and even more.

This exercise should always be done on an empty stomach, before breakfast. This posture helps in elimination of waste products. It also strengthens the abdominal muscles. On the whole, it is an excellent pose and should be practiced by everyone, daily, in the morning, especially by persons suffering from constipation.

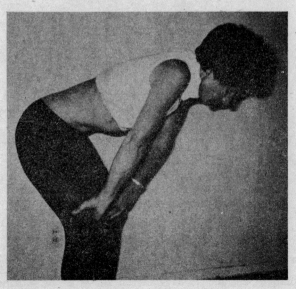

Figure 21–1   Josette Guerne

Arm Circling Exercise

I. a. Stand with legs slightly apart. Place both hands, palms down on your solar plexus.

   b. Inhale, raising your right arm up until it is high above the head, eyes following the movement of the arm (Figure 22–1).

   c. Exhale, bringing the right hand down and raising the left simultaneously. Repeat five times, circling around with one arm. It should be done rhythmically, slowly, and gracefully. Then bring both hands back to the solar plexus.

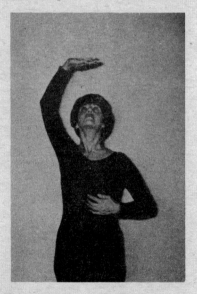

Figure 22–1 Phyllis Sampson

II. a. Inhale and slowly circle both arms up above your head, fingers of both hands meeting. Eyes up. Hold briefly.

    b. Exhale, circling arms gracefully down to the starting position, hands back on the solar plexus. Repeat a few times.

This is a very soothing posture and it has a wonderful calming influence on the nervous system and on the whole being. My students call it "cosmic breathing." Try it whenever you feel tired or nervous and see what happens.

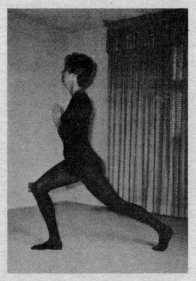

Figure 23–1   Ann Dunn

Spine Exercise

a.   Take a long step, palms together on the chest, the upper part of the body straight.

b.   Inhale, bending the right knee, the left leg stretched out (Figure 23–1). Hold for five seconds.

c.   Exhale, bringing the leg back to starting position. Alternate three or four times.

This is good for the posture and the spine.

Triangle Pose—Trikonasan

I. a. Place legs well apart and arms stretched sideways.
   b. Inhale in this position.
   c. Exhale, bending to the right foot (Figure 24–1).
   d. Hold briefly and return to standing position. Alternate, and
      repeat three times.

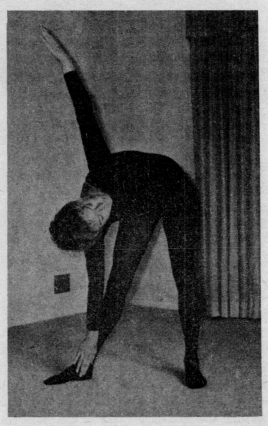

Figure 24–1   Ann Dunn

II. Variation
   a. Remain in standing position, arms stretched.
   b. Inhale, twisting the body, right arm first. Head turns in the same direction.
   c. Exhale, and slowly bend, right hand touching left foot, and left hand straight out (Figure 24–2). Alternate, and repeat five times.

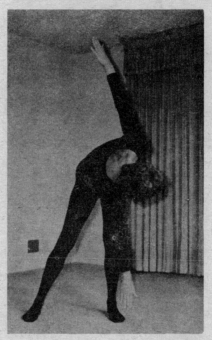

Figure 24–2   Ann Dunn

Both of these postures tone the spinal nerves and the abdominal organs. They also stretch the muscles and keep the spine elastic. Good for everyone. But start slowly to begin with until you are sure that the muscles are flexible and no strain will be felt on the back.

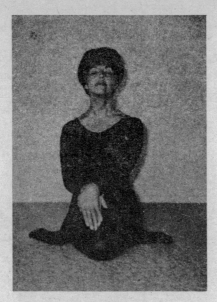

Figure 25–1   Phyllis Sampson

THIRD WEEK

The Bull's Face

a.   Sit in a squatting position.

b.   Bend both knees and place one on top of the other.

c.   Sit on your heels with toes out. Place hands on top of the knees, one on top of the other, spine perfectly straight, eyes closed (Figure 25–1).

d.   Now you can do deep breathing, and remain in this pose as long as you feel comfortable.

Push-Ups Exercise

a.   Lie stretched out, feet together, hands along the body.

b.   Inhale, lifting head and feet (about six inches) off the floor (Figure 26–1).

c.   Exhale, as you lie down to starting pose. Repeat three times.

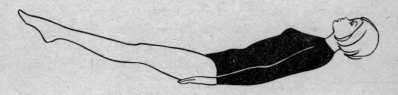

Figure 26–1

This posture is excellent to strengthen stomach muscles. It also stretches the spinal cord.

Abdominal Stretch Exercise

I. a. Lie flat on the floor.
   b. Place feet together, arms along the body.
   c. Inhale, raising the right leg and the left arm, simultaneously (Figure 27–1).
   d. Exhale, return to starting position. Alternate, and repeat five times.

II.   Variation
   a. Remain in the same position flat on the floor.
   b. Inhale, raising both legs and both arms, simultaneously, arms to shoulder level (Figure 27–2).
   c. Exhale, and sink slowly to starting position. Repeat three times.

This posture firms the chest or bust. It also strengthens the stomach muscles and reduces the hips.

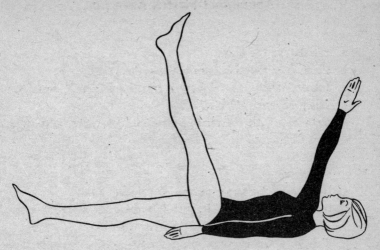

Figure 27-1

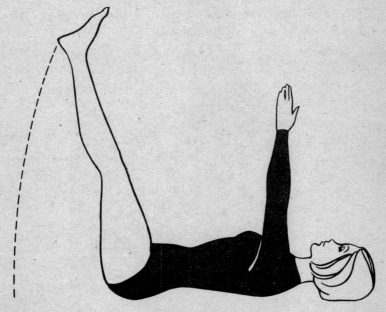

Figure 27-2

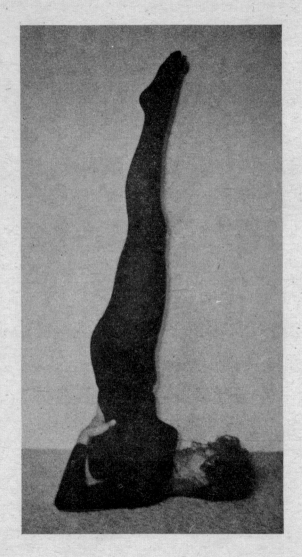

Figure 28–1   Ann Dunn

Shoulderstand—Sarvangasan

a. Lie flat on the back. Start slowly raising both legs, and then lift the trunk and hips.
b. Rest elbows on the floor, hands supporting the back.
c. Legs should be absolutely vertical, chin pressed against the chest (Figure 28-1).
d. Keep breathing in this position, slowly and deeply, and try to remain in it as long as you feel comfortable. Start with one minute and then increase to five and later even to ten.
e. While you are in this position, you can do some bicycling with your legs. Then come down slowly, without jerky movements.

Shoulderstand should be practiced by the student who feels that the muscles have limbered up. It is considered an advanced posture. It is also suggested when in this pose try to concentrate on the thyroid glands, situated in the neck. This posture has ·a tremendous impact on all parts of the body. It has a rejuvenating effect on the whole system, too. It helps promote the secretion of the thyroid, which is one of the major glands of the endocrine system. By reversing the position, an additional supply of blood is brought to the thyroid which in turn helps to promote the functioning of other parts of the body.
The Yogis considered that this posture would keep wrinkles away. It is also of great help to nervous conditions, since additional blood and oxygen are brought to the spinal column.

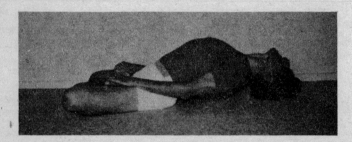

Figure 29–3　　Tom Abbott

Fish Posture—Matsyasan

a.　Lie flat on the back.

b.　Prop the body up on elbows, legs stretched out, for beginners. More advanced students keep legs in Lotus position (Figure 29–1).

c.　Rest the crown of the head on the floor.

d.　Hold this position for at least 30 seconds, increasing with time, and breathe rhythmically in and out, through the nose.

This position relieves cramps in the neck. It also brings blood and oxygen into the thyroid and parathyroid glands, stimulating their functions. These glands play a vital part in the physiological functioning of the various systems of the body. The abdominal muscles are exercised, too.

Head-Knee Pose—Paschimathan Asana

a.   Stretch on the floor on your back, arms above the head, also stretched.

b.   Inhale, slowly raising the head and chest and assume a sitting position.

c.   Exhale, continuing to bend the body until you are able to catch the toes of your feet. Your face should be buried between the knees (Figure 30-1). Hold briefly. Repeat this exercise three times.

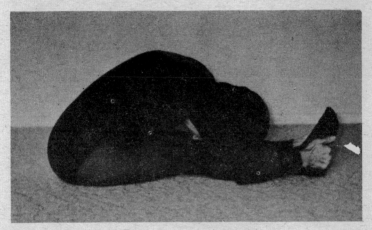

Figure 30-1   Phyllis Sampson

This exercise stimulates the kidneys, liver and pancreas. The knees strengthen, too, as the posture should be done with knees absolutely straight. It also has a rejuvenating effect on the whole system. By keeping the head low, the facial muscles get an additional supply of blood and oxygen.

It is a good idea after the Paschimathan Asana to get into the Supine pose (which follows), to stretch the spine into the opposite direction.

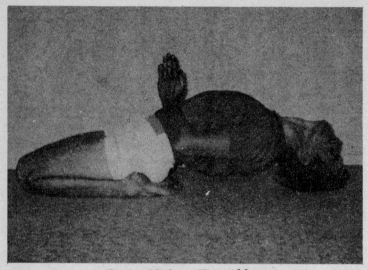

Figure 31–1   Tom Abbott

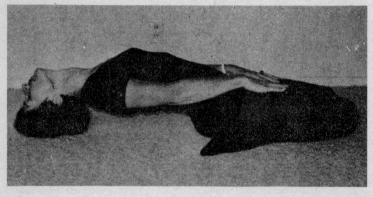

Figure 31–2   Phyllis Sampson

Supine Pose

a.   Sit on your heels.
b.   Then stretch backwards, slowly.
c.   Let the head fall back, resting on the floor.
d.   The spine is off the floor, palms together on the chest (Figure 31–1).
e.   Hold this position while doing the deep rhythmic breathing.
f.   (Figure 31–2) shows a different way of holding the hands.
g.   Here the same posture is demonstrated by a twelve-year-old boy (Figure 31–3).

This posture is excellent for stretching the spine, but also the stretching is felt in the upper legs. It keeps the neck smooth from wrinkles and has a rejuvenating effect on the facial muscles.

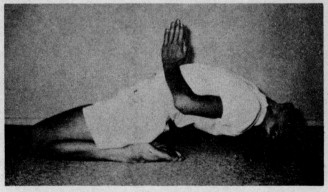

Figure 31–3   Chris Dunn

Cobra Pose—Bhujangasan

a)   Lie flat on the stomach, chin on the floor, elbows out and
     both hands next to the chin (Figure 32–1), completely
     relaxed.
b)   Inhale, raising the upper part of the body slowly off the
     floor (Figure 32–2), spine well arched.
c)   Hold your breath for a few seconds, keeping head up and
     backwards, as far as possible.
d)   Exhale and return to starting position. Repeat three times.
     Relax.

This posture helps to remove tension, and it keeps the spine
strong and flexible. It should relieve any back discomfort. Feel
every vertebrae bending, one by one, as you raise the body. It
brings life to the spine.
This posture also helps to strengthen abdominal muscles and
tone them due to the stretching of the upper part of the body.
The Cobra pose is very beneficial to women, as it tones the
female organs. It is also a beautifying exercise as by stretching
the neck it keeps it smooth, free from wrinkles, naturally giving
it a much younger appearance.

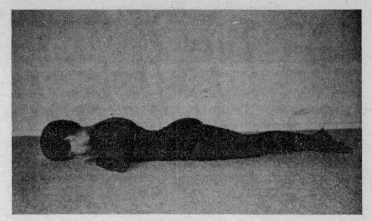

Figure 32–1

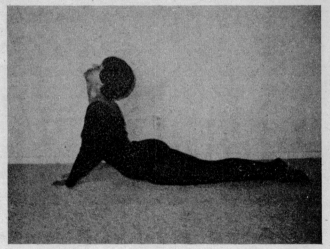

Figure 32–2

Phyllis Sampson

Half-Locust Pose—Arhda-Salabhasan

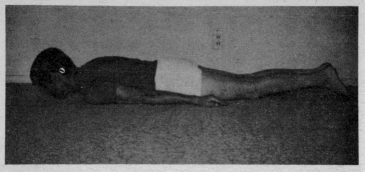

Figure 33–1   Tom Abbott

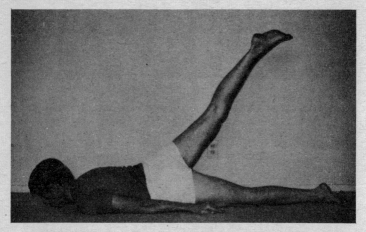

Figure 33–2

a.   Lie flat on the abdomen, chin on the floor, hands at sides (Figure 33–1).

b.   Inhale, raising the right leg as high as possible away from the floor (Figures 33–2). Hold your breath for a few seconds in this position.

c.   Exhale and slowly bring the leg down to starting position.

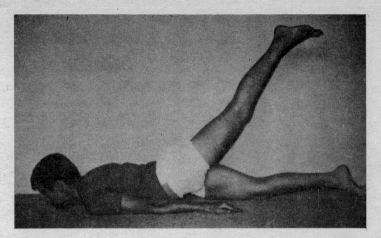

Tom Abbott

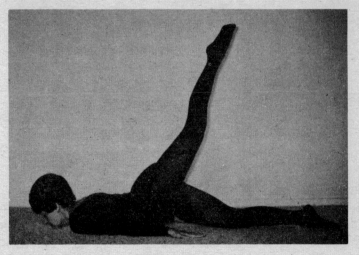

Figure 33–3 Phyllis Sampson

d. Alternate, doing the same with the left leg (Figure 33–3). Repeat at least three times with each leg, and practice the Half-Locust pose before you attempt to try the Full-Locust pose.

Full-Locust Pose—Salabhasan

a.   Resume the same starting position as for the *Half-Locust Pose*.

b.   Place both fists under the thighs, chin on the floor.

c.   Inhale and lift both legs, simultaneously, pushing yourself up (Figure 34–1).

d.   Holding breath briefly, remaining in this position.

e.   Exhale and bring legs slowly down to the floor. Repeat it twice.

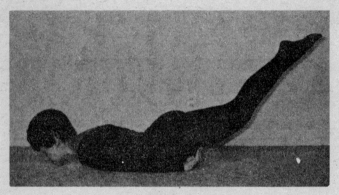

Figure 34–1   Phyllis Sampson

Full-Locust pose should be practiced after the student has accomplished the Half-Locust with ease. In the Full-Locust the force is put on your hands and on your chin, too, to be able to lift the body. It is an excellent exercise for your back, as it exerts a pressure on the back muscles, thus increasing the blood circulation.

Rolling Exercise

a. Lie flat on your back, arms above the head.
b. Link your thumbs.
c. Inhale, rolling to the right, raising feet and arms simultaneously (Figure 35–1).
d. Exhale, rolling over to the other side.

This is good for the joints and for the spine.

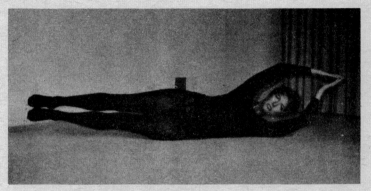

Figure 35–1   Ann Dunn

Spinal Stretch—Paschimothan Asana

a. Lie stretched out flat on the floor, both arms stretched above the head.
b. Inhale, slowly raising both legs and both arms, simultaneously. Try to reach the feet with your fingers (Figure 36–1). Hold briefly.
c. Exhale, and return to starting position. Repeat twice.

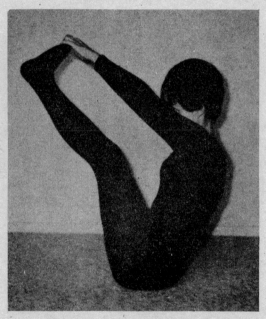

Figure 36–1   Phyllis Sampson

This posture is very good for the leg muscles, also for abdominal muscles. It has a rejuvenating effect on the whole body. It also stretches the spine.

FOURTH WEEK

Leg Exercises

I. a. Lie on the right side, resting the head on the arm, the other hand on the floor (Figure 37–1).
   b. Inhale, lifting the leg as high as possible, and as comfortably as you can.
   c. Hold for five seconds, holding your breath (Figure 37–2).
   d. Exhale, and bring the leg to starting position. Repeat five times.

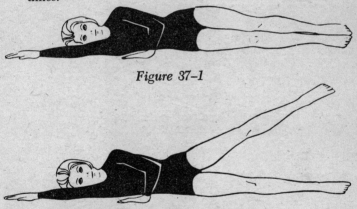

Figure 37–1

Figure 37–2

II. a. Remaining in the same position, bring the leg forward and then backwards. Inhale, as you move forward, and exhale, as you bring the leg backwards. Repeat five times.

   b. You can add variety by first bringing the leg forward, then up, and then backwards. First inhale as you bring leg forward, hold your breath as you raise the leg, and exhale as you move it backwards.

These exercises help to stretch the leg muscles and keep you in good shape.

III. a. Lie stretched out on the floor on the back, arms along the body (Figure 38–1).

    b. Inhale, bringing the leg straight up (Figure 38–2).

    c. Hold your breath for five seconds, simultaneously bringing the leg over the thigh sideways (Figure 38–3) and up again.

Figure 38–1   Phyllis Sampson

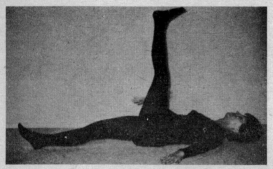

Figure 38–2

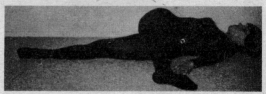

Figure 38–3

    d. Now exhale, and lower the leg to starting position.

    e. Reverse the posture, doing the same with the other leg. Repeat three times.

This exercise stretches the thigh and hip muscles.

Cat Pose

a. Kneel on hands and knees (Figure 39–1).
b. Inhale deeply and rhythmically, humping your back, and
    bringing the right knee toward the face, lowering face to
    meet the knee in slow motion (Figure 39–2).

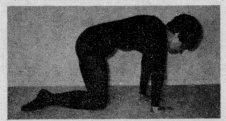

Figure 39–1 Phyllis Sampson

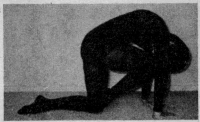

Figure 39–2

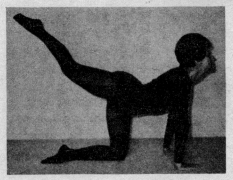

Figure 39–3

c. Holding your breath, lift right leg as far as you can com-
    fortably, without strain or pull, away from the body
    (Figure 39–3). Do it slowly and gracefully.

d. Exhale, and bring the knee down to starting position as demonstrated in (Figure 39–1).

e. Alternate, following the same method. Repeat at least three times and increase the number to five as time goes on.

f. Relax for a while and follow up with the *Cat Stretch*.

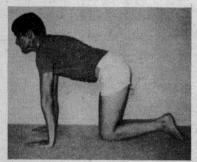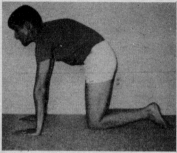

Figure 39–1 Tom Abbott

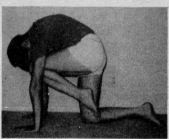

Figure 39–2

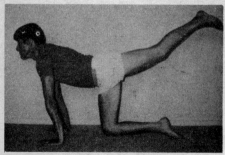

Figure 39–3

Cat Stretch Pose

a.   Assume the same starting position as in the Cat pose (Figure 40–1).

b.   Hump your back (Figure 40–2).

c.   Inhale rhythmically, then slowly and gracefully sit down on your heels (Figure 40–3).

d.   Holding your breath, slide forward, face close to the floor (Figure 40–4).

e.   Exhale and slowly raise the body to starting position as in (Figure 40–1). Repeat three times, and relax, resuming (Figure 40–3) and continue to do the deep breathing.

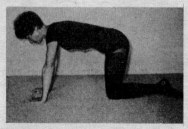

Figure 40–1   Ann Dunn

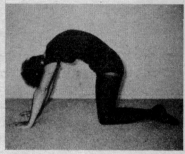

Figure 40–2

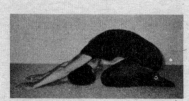

Figure 40–3

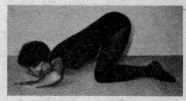

Figure 40–4

Both exercises, the Cat pose and the Cat stretch pose are very beneficial for the female organs. It releases the pressure and stimulates the gonad (or sex) glands. Simultaneously, it works on our back, arms and shoulders, making it stronger by giving an additional stretch and pull. Of course, any of these postures bring additional oxygen into our system, stimulating the blood and purifying it. As long as the face, head and neck assume a position down, the circulation firms the muscles of the neck, the jaw, and the facial muscles. All together, it keeps the wrinkles away in the face and in the neck.

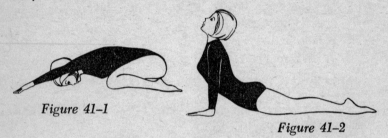

Figure 41–1

Figure 41–2

Swan Pose

a. Sit on your heels.
b. Bend the head down, stretching arms forward as far as you can, face touching the floor (Figure 41–1).
c. Inhale, come forward, into the Cobra pose, resting on your arms (Figure 41–2). Hold for five to ten seconds.
d. Exhale, and come back to starting position slowly and gracefully.

In this posture the spine stretches both ways. Benefits derived from this posture are similar to the Cobra pose. It stimulates the function around the pelvic region and the abdominal muscles are at work, too.

It is advisable to remain in starting position (Figure 41–1) for a while, breathing deeply and rhythmically. This brings blood and additional oxygen to your brain. Besides, it is a good relaxing pose.

Spinal Twist Pose—Ardha-Matsyendrasan

a. Sit with legs stretched out.
b. Then bend the left leg at the knee and set the heel against the thigh.
c. Now bend the right leg at the knee and rest over the external side of the thigh.
d. Beginners can simplify the posture holding the right ankle with the left hand. Right hand resting on the back (Figure 42–1).
e. More advanced students would slightly change the pose, by passing the left arm over the right knee, and catch the right ankle as in (Figure 42–2).

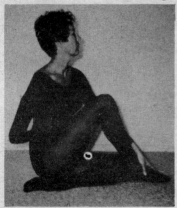

Figure 42–1 Ann Dunn

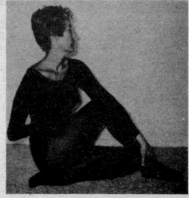

Figure 42–2

f.   Inhale, sitting in this position before you start turning your neck and shoulders, simultaneously. Chest erect, chin up (Figure 42–3) forms the complete pose.

g.   Hold for five seconds and return to starting position. Repeat a few times, and then alternate the same pose, using the same technique.

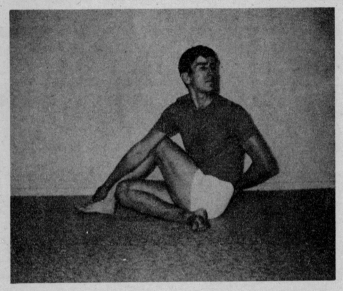

Figure 42–3   Tom Abbott in complete pose.

The Twist has many benefits. It keeps the spine elastic. Besides, the spinal nerves are toned by the rich supply of blood and oxygen. It also massages the abdominal organs and helps with constipation. Muscular rheumatism can be helped due to twisting the spine, for the circulation increases, which in turn can relieve pain and discomfort. In addition, this pose massages the kidneys, thus it is important to practice it daily.

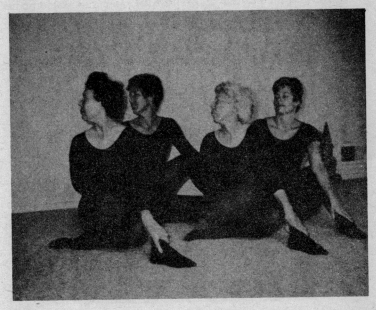

A group of my students in the class doing the Twist (Figure 42–5).

Sideway Swing Exercise

a. Sit on floor, knees drawn to one side, hands clasped above the head (Figure 43-1).

b. Inhale, sitting in this position.

c. Then exhale, swinging to the side (Figure 43-2).

d. Reverse the position and repeat the same. Suggested about three times on each side.

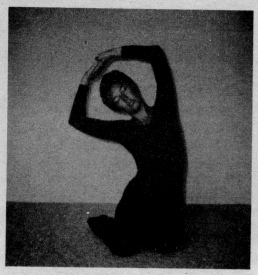

Figure 43-1   Ann Dunn

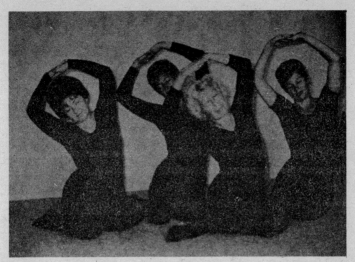

Figure 43-2   Roxy Reed, Ann Dunn, Jessie Agena, Marsha Carr

The Swing helps to reduce the waistline and also stimulates the functioning of the liver and spleen. It should be included in your daily routine, after you have advanced with your program. Students favor this pose very much and like to practice it in groups.

Standing Exercises for Good Posture and Balance

I. a. Stand upright with outstretched arms.
   b. Bend knees as though you are about to sit down on a chair (Figure 44–1). Inhale doing it.
   c. Then exhale, returning to upright position. Repeat twice.

This stimulates kidney function.

II. a. Stand on your toes, lifting arms above the head.
    b. Inhale, stretching as far as you can (Figure 44–2).
    c. Exhale, and return to standing position. Repeat three times.

This is excellent for the spine.

III. a. Stand on your left leg, the right toes around the ankle.
     b. Inhale, lifting left heel up, standing on your toes (Figure 44–3).
     c. Exhale, getting down to starting position.
     d. Reverse the posture, and do the same with the other leg. Repeat four times with each leg.

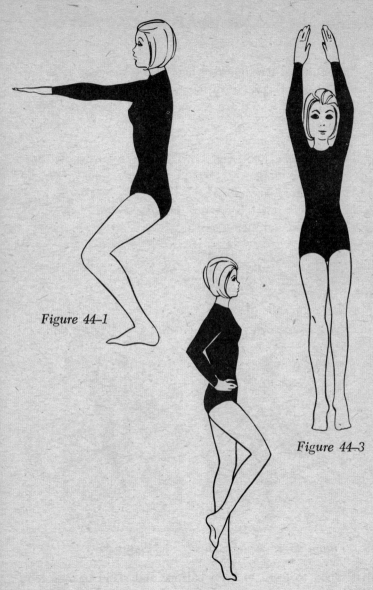

Figure 44-1

Figure 44-2

Figure 44-3

The Stork Pose

a.   Stand erect, the right foot bent at the knee and raised up to the left thigh. Grasp toes with left hand.

b.   Place right arm above the head, well stretched (Figure 45–1).

c.   Inhale, standing in this position.

d.   Then exhale, and bend down, trying to reach the floor with your fingers. It should be done slowly, without forcing it (Figure 45–2).

e.   Hold for a few seconds and increase to ten seconds. Repeat twice and then alternate.

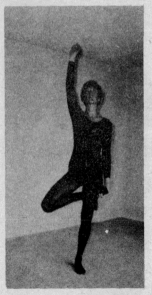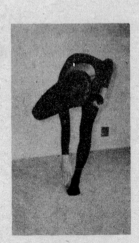

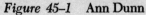

Figure 45–1   Ann Dunn   *Figure 45–2*

This is good to learn to keep balance and stand on one foot. At the same time it does stretch the spine and brings blood to the head and facial muscles.

The Tree Pose—Trishasan

a.   Stand with feet apart.
b.   Bend the right knee and let the foot sole rest on the left thigh.
c.   Stretch arms above the head, palms together (Figure 46-1). Inhale.
d.   Hold for a few seconds, or as long as you can. Then exhale, and bring the leg to starting position.
e.   Alternate. Repeat two or three times.
f.   The advanced student should try the same pose, but slowly rise on toes.

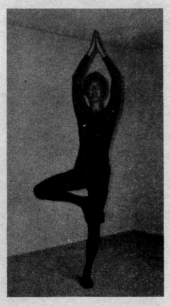

Figure 46-1   Ann Dunn

This teaches balance, but it is also beneficial for the entire nervous system, as it has a rejuvenating effect on the body.

Lord Matarajasan Pose

a. First stand up straight. Left arm stretched.
b. Raise the right foot backwards and bend the knee. Grasp the right ankle with the right hand, and pull ankle back (Figure 47–1).
c. Inhale, pulling the leg away as far as you can (Figures 47–2 and 47–3).
d. Exhale, returning to standing position. Alternate.

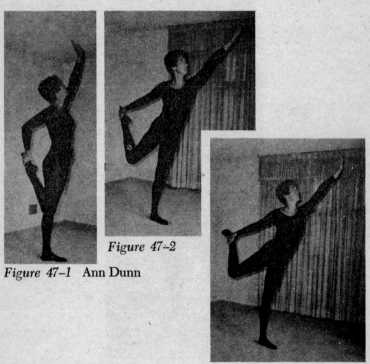

Figure 47–2

Figure 47–1   Ann Dunn

Figure 47–3

This exercise stretches various ligaments and also the leg muscles. It is also an excellent way to keep balance.

The Moon Posture—Chandrasana

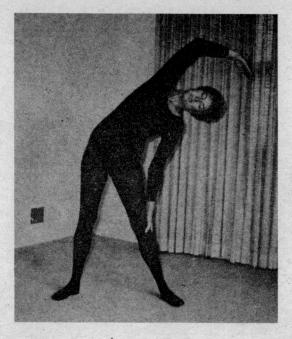

Figure 48–1

a.   Stand straight, knees firm, arms along the body.

b.   Inhale, stretching arms sideways and placing legs wide apart.

c.   Then exhale, bending to the left side from the waist up, right arm over the head, and left holding on to your knee (Figure 48–1).

d.   Return to starting position and repeat the same to the other side.

This posture helps to reduce the waistline. It also helps stretch the spinal muscles. It is very soothing to the whole nervous system.

ADVANCED YOGA

Salute to the Sun—Soorya Namaskar

This exercise should be practiced in the morning. In the earlier days, the Yogis practiced this daily, as it combines various postures and it helps to limber up.

a. Stand straight, hands folded in front of the chest, legs together. Try to face the sun (Figure 49–1).

b. Inhale deeply and rhythmically. Raise the hands, and bend backwards as far as you can comfortably. Don't strain at any time (Figure 49–2).

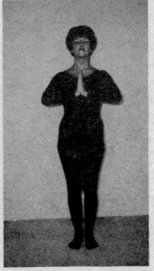 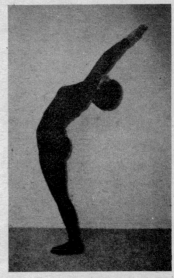

Figure 49–1   Phyllis Sampson   Figure 49–2

c.   Now start exhaling, bending forward till your hands reach
     the feet. The head should touch the knees and the knees
     should be straight (Figure 49–3). However, until you
     limber up, you can slightly bend the knees.
d.   Inhale deeply, keeping hands on the floor, left knee bent
     and right leg moved away from the body, head raised up
     (Figure 49–4).

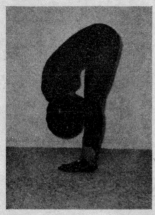

Figure 49–3

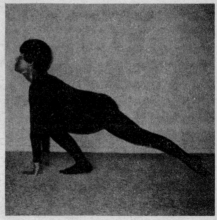

Figure 49–4

e. Hold your breath, placing both feet away from the body and raise the body off the floor, supported by hands and toes (Figure 49–5).

f. Exhaling, bring the knees to the floor first, then curve the spine and lower the face (Figure 49–6).

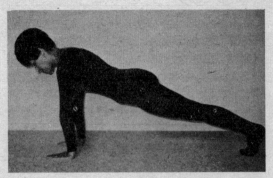

Figure 49–5

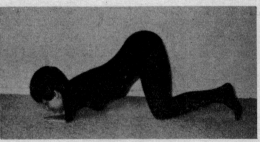

Figure 49–6

g. Inhale, and bend the upper part of the body backwards, legs back, similar to the Cobra pose, face upwards (Figure 49–7).

h. Now exhale, lifting the body up, but keep the heels and hands firmly on the floor (Figure 49–8).

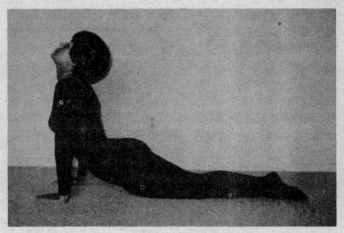

Figure 49–7

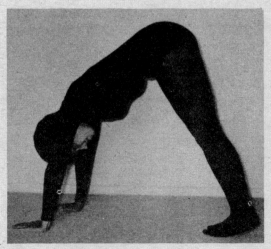

Figure 49–8

i.   Inhale, bringing the right foot toward the hands, while left foot and knee should go backwards and touch the ground, head and face upwards (Figure 49–9).

j.   Exhale, bringing the left leg forward, knees straight again, head as close as possible to the knees (Figure 49–10).

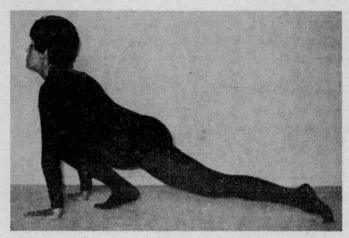

Figure 49–11

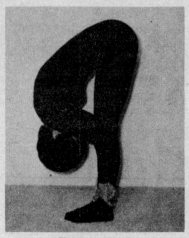

Figure 49–12

k.   Inhale, bending backwards, raising the hands and the head (Figure 49–11).

l.   Exhale, bringing hands together as in the starting position (Figure 49–12).

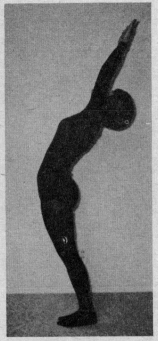

Figure 49–9

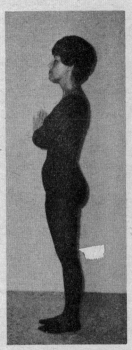

Figure 49–10

These postures are a combination of various movements which will improve flexibility of the spine and limbs. They also reduce the abdomen, and waistline. The combination of postures and deep breathing promotes the blood circulation.

All twelve positions make one exercise. It should be repeated at least three times in the beginning, and slowly increase to ten times daily. It takes in every part of the body.

Forward Roll Exercise

a.   Kneel, keeping knees and arms close, spine round.

b.   Place the crown of the head on the floor and roll slightly forward (Figure 50–1).

c.   Inhale, as you place the head down, and then exhale, and sit down on your heels.

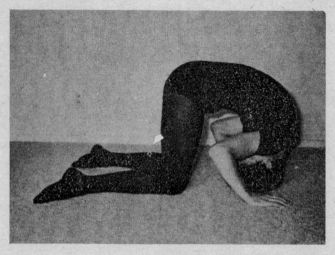

Figure 50–1

This pose brings additional blood and oxygen to the brain, and it also has a rejuvenating effect on facial muscles and the skin.

Kneeling Pose

a. Kneel, keeping body straight and arms folded around the shoulders (Figure 51-1).

b. Inhale, turning to the far right (Figure 51-2).

c. Hold your breath and bend your body to the floor, making a complete circle (Figures 51-3 and 51-4).

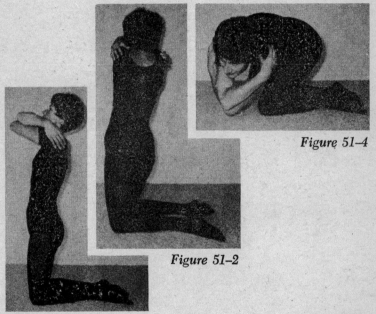

Figure 51-4

Figure 51-2

Figure 51-1 Josette Guerne

Figure 51-3

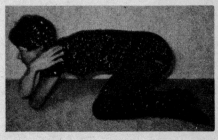

d.   Exhale, lift the body up and turn to the extreme left.

e.   And now with a fast jerk bring your arms and body to the far right, to the same point from where you have started. Repeat about three times.

This is an excellent posture to get any discomfort out of the neck, or help a stiff neck.

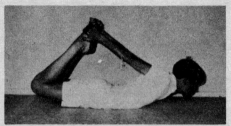

Figure 52–1 Chris Dunn

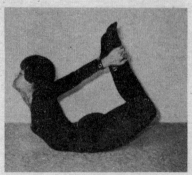

Figure 52–2 Phyllis Sampson

Bow Pose—Dhanurasan

a.   Lie flat on your stomach, bend the legs.

b.   Catch the right ankle with the right hand, and the left with the left hand, chin on the floor (Figure 52–1).

c. Inhale, lifting the whole body and head (Figure 52–2).
d. Advanced students should rock forward and backwards.
e. Exhale and return to starting position. Relax. Repeat twice.

This pose is the combination of the Cobra and Locust exercises. The back muscles are well involved in this posture. Doing it daily will reduce fat and relieve any congestion of the blood in the abdominal viscera. It is specially recommended for women.

Plough Pose—Halasan

a. Lie flat on your back, hands at your sides, palms down (Figure 53–1).
b. Inhaling, raise the legs (Figure 53–2).

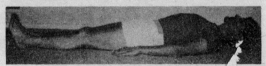

Figure 53–1   Tom Abbott

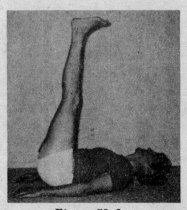

Figure 53–2

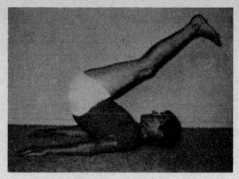

Figure 53–3

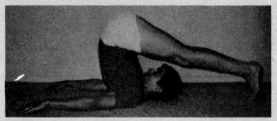

Figure 53–4

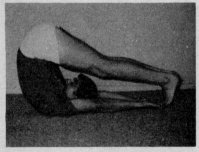

Figure 53–5

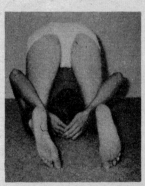

Figure 53–5

c.   Then slowly raise the hips without bending the legs (Figure 53–3).

d.   Continue raising the body until the toes touch the floor (Figure 53–4), knees and feet together.

e.   Now move your arms toward the feet and with palms up touch the toes. Keep knees absolutely straight (Figure 53–5).

f.   Hold for a few seconds. Then exhale and bring the body slowly, without any jerking movements, to starting position as in (Figure 53–1) and then relax.

g.   Before returning to starting position, you can finish the Plough Pose with a further step with the knees and arms bent toward the floor on both sides of the ears. This pose by itself it called the Ear-Knee pose or in Sanskrit, Karna Peedasan. To return to starting position roll slowly forward, again without jerky movements.

This posture gives an additional stretch to the whole spine. Every vertebra receives additional blood. It is vital to good health to keep the spine limber and flexible. All kinds of bendings of the spine are effective to the abdominal muscles and should be done repeatedly to keep in perfect condition. In the beginning these exercises might seem difficult, but as you go on practicing it is much easier to do them.

Good posture and a flexible spine contribute much to better health and through daily exercises of yoga anyone can greatly improve any imperfection in that particular region. A flexible spine gives a youthful appearance no matter what the calendar age. A straight spine looks young and a curved one gives an impression of a tired feeling and old age. By doing the yoga exercises you can prevent from accumulating the abnormal mineral deposits in the bones. Due to better blood circulation and additional oxygen to purify the blood, the condition of these deposits can be greatly improved.

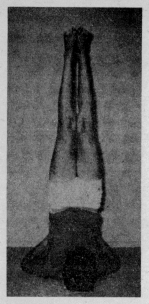

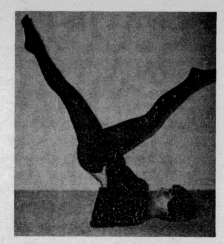

Figure 54–2 Phyllis Sampson

Figure 54–1   Tom Abbott

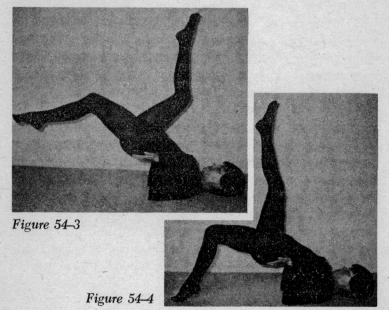

Figure 54–3

Figure 54–4

Bridge Pose—Sethu Bandhasana

a. After you have mastered the shoulderstand and feel comfortable in its pose (Figure 54-1), try to come down lowering one leg at a time to the floor in front (Figures 54-2 and 54-3).

b. Arms support the back with fingers around the waistline or on hips (Figure 54-4).

c. Finally, both feet will rest on the floor (Figure 54-5).

d. Inhale, remaining in this position for five to ten seconds or even longer, if you feel comfortable.

e. Exhale, raising your legs to resume the shoulderstand pose again. Repeat twice, increasing the number later on.

This posture is for fairly advanced students. It stretches every part of the body. But don't attempt to do it unless you are flexible and feel you are ready for it.

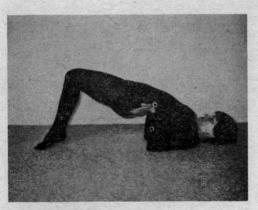

Figure 54-5

Wheel Pose—Chakrasana

a. Lie down on the floor, bend the knees, bring arms behind the head, palms down on the floor (Figure 55–1).

b. Inhale, raising the body as high as possible, bending the spine (Figure 55–2).

c. Continue to raise body until your spin is well rounded and the head, if possible, off the floor (Figure 55–3).

d. Hold your breath for five to ten seconds. Then exhale and return to starting position. Repeat twice.

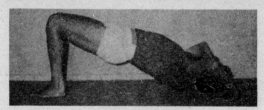

Figure 55–1   Tom Abbott

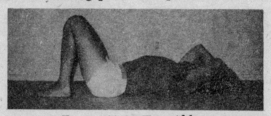

Figure 55–2

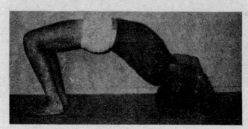

Figure 55–3

In this asana the muscles of the legs, hips, spine and arms get a perfect stretching and bending.

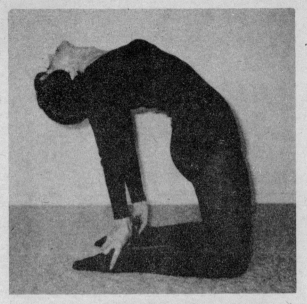

Figure 56–1   Phyllis Sampson

Pelvic Stretch Pose

a. Kneel, stretch arms.
b. Inhale, and clasp ankles with your hands, and bend head as far as possible (Figure 56–1).
c. Hold for a while.
d. Then exhale and return to starting position. Repeat this exercise two to three times.

This firms up the hips and thighs and stretches the neck. It brings additional circulation into the thyroid glands.

Exercises to Strengthen the Pelvic Region

I. a. Lie on your back, raising legs with straight knees about six inches from the floor, arms stretched out (Figure 57–1).
   b. Inhale, moving legs to the left, heels together, knees together. Keep the upper body flat on the floor (Figure 57–2).
   c. Exhale, moving in the same way to the right.
   d. Return to starting position and repeat four times.

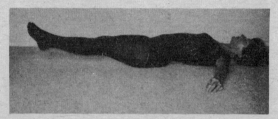

Figure 57–1

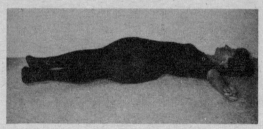

Figure 57–2   Josette Guerne

II. a. Lie flat on the floor, bend the knees (Figure 57–3).
    b. Inhale, turning the knees to the left, keeping them off the floor (Figure 57–4).
    c. Exhale, stretching legs out (Figure 57–5).
    d. Bring legs around to the right still stretched out and inhale deeply.
    e. Exhale and bend the knees.
    f. Return to starting position and repeat three times.

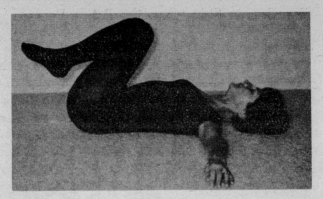

Figure 57-3

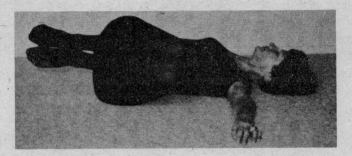

Figure 57-4

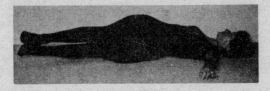

Figure 57-5

This exercise is helpful to tone up the abdominal muscles as well as bring better circulation to the legs from hip down. It looks simple, but if it is done properly it is quite strenuous and should not be attempted by a beginner.

Headstand Pose—Sirshasan

The Headstand is called king of yoga postures. It acts as a tonic to the whole nervous system. The extra blood supply sent to the brain stimulates the endocrine glands situated there. But the Headstand should not be attempted without a doctor's consent by anyone who has a weak neck, spine, or any other discomfort. It should not be done by persons with high blood pressure or thyroid deficiency. It is a very beneficial exercise, but can be harmful if done by a person at the wrong time. After you have practiced the other exercises for a while and feel that you have made some progress, then try the Headstand, but do not try it from the start. Begin doing it for 30 seconds and slowly increase your time to about five minutes a day. Do not stand on your head any longer than that unless you have practiced yoga for many years and have become very good at it. Before you attempt to do the Headstand, it is important to be able to relax your body completely.

a. Arms, elbows and hands are used for support. Kneel down on a soft carpet. Interlock the fingers and place hands on the floor with little fingers down. Place elbows on the floor on both sides of the ears. Put your head down and, about one inch above your forehead, place it in the hollow of your palms. Make sure you are comfortable (Figure 58–1).

b. Raise your legs slowly (Figure 58–2).

c. Now start walking on the toes toward your torso, until your spine is perfectly straight.

d. Now slowly start raising legs, knees bent (Figure 58–3).

e. Continue to raise straight up, with spine absolutely straight (Figure 58–4).

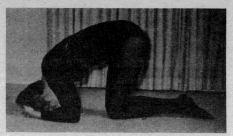

Figure 58–1   Ann Dunn

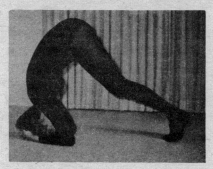

Figure 58–2

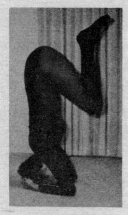

Figure 58–3

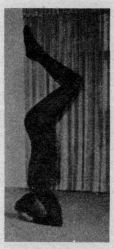

Figure 58–4

f. Finally rise to the last stretch when the body will be straight from toes to head. Make sure that you are comfortable and there is no strain on your head. Do rhythmic breathing while standing on your head (Figure 58–5). Keep eyes closed and relax.

g. To come down, use the same method, reversing the positions. It should be done slowly, without jerky movements and with concentration.

h. Finish by sitting on your heels, hands stretched out, and take a deep breath (Figure 58–6). During the headstand blood rushes into the head, and by reversing the position of the head rapidly you might get a feeling of dizziness. Thus to avoid dizziness, it is essential to finish in this position.

There is still another way to practice the headstand. Until you have the necessary balance to stand on your head in the middle of the room, use a wall or corner of the room. Use the same method as previously explained. The distance between your hands and the wall should be approximately the length of the arms from wrist to elbow. It is a good idea, at first, to have someone to help you to bring one leg up next to the wall. After that, you will be able to bring up the other one without difficulties. Hold the position for about thirty seconds. Then bend the knees and begin to lower your legs, one at a time, slowly, until your toes touch the floor. It is important to do this exercise slowly and not hurt yourself by fast motions. Finish the same way as above with hands stretched out, taking a deep breath.

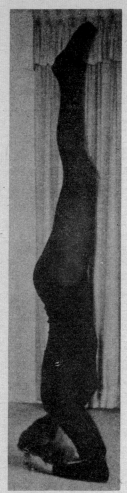

Figure 58–5

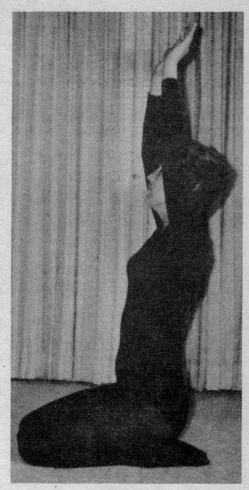

Figure 58–6

Boat Pose

a. Lie flat on the floor, arms extended.
b. Inhale, and raise both legs and arms off the floor (Figure 59-1). Hold briefly.
c. Exhale and bring the body down to the floor. Repeat several times.

This is excellent for the spine and the benefits are similar to the ones derived when you practice the Lotus pose.

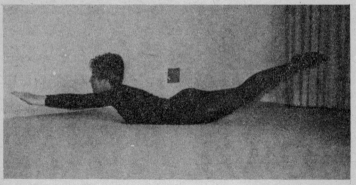

Figure 59–1   Ann Dunn

Flying Pose

a. Lie flat on the floor, extending arms sideways, like wings of an airplane.
b. Inhale and raise your upper and lower body up as high as you can comfortably (Figure 60–1). Hold briefly.
c. Exhale, bringing the body down to the floor. Repeat several times.

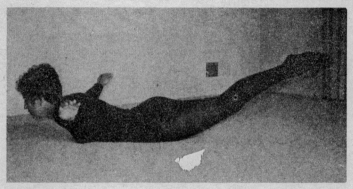

Figure 60–1

Perfect-Balance Pose

a.   Stand on one leg, raising the other backward straight with the body. Place one hand along the thigh and the other in front of your chin (Figure 61–1). Inhale. Hold briefly.

b.   Exhale and bring the leg down. Alternate with the other leg. Repeat several times.

The student who can stand on one leg perfectly straight, has accomplished a balance of the body.

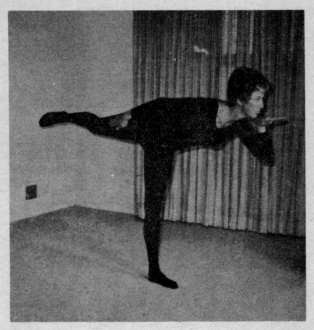

Figure 61–1

TOM ABBOTT

One day Tom Abbott came to my studio with the idea that he would like to study yoga. He had little knowledge of it, but he wanted to find the answer to how he could improve his mental and physical conditions. He had heard that yoga might help. At that time, he seemed quite nervous, impatient and very negative.

I invited him to join some of my classes. When he appeared at the first class, conducted at the Alondra Park, in Lawndale, California, one of my schools, I suggested that he get down to the floor and follow the others, but he was dubious. "I could never do these things," he said. It was an advanced group of students who had studied for quite a while with me.

Nevertheless, I ignored his statement and suggested he get down on the floor and try his best. Indeed, he was stiff and clumsy, but the others did not pay attention to him. In the yoga class, everyone is busy with his own work and doesn't pay much attention to others, unless someone is asking for help. In class, I suggest keeping the eyes closed, so your neighbor won't feel embarrassed.

Dubious, but fascinated by the others who looked so much at ease in the various positions, Tom, too, began to follow the class and forget his shortcomings. In fact, he was enthralled and I began to see improvements by the second lesson, a week later. Shortly afterwards, he inquired whether he could join another class to have an opportunity to study more. I suggested a class at my private studio, where smaller groups form a class, and where I would be able to watch him closer and correct his mistakes.

Six months later, Tom Abbott was able to do the most difficult yoga posture gracefully and with great ease. His nerves calmed down and he now looks at life with a different approach. Not only has he become a very advanced student, but he also became interested in teaching, to share with others what he has learned in such a short time.

I was glad to welcome Tom Abbott to my staff of assistants, as he so well understands the problem of the many people who come to our studio for help, however dubious and negative they are about the results. One must give one's mind a chance to find out the truth, and give one's body the opportunity to experience the results, before one says no.

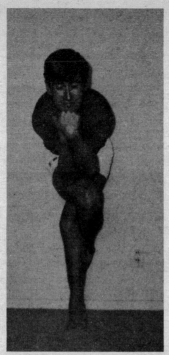

Figure 62–1   Tom Abbott

Eagle Pose—Garuda Asana

a.   Stand upright. The left leg is slightly bent. The right leg wound around it. Bend forward and get the arms into the same position as the legs. The chin rests on the back of the hand (Figure 62–1). Remain in this pose for a while doing your deep breathing. Then alternate.

Peacock Pose—Mayoorasan

a.   Kneel on the floor.

b.   Rest the hands on the floor with palms down and fingers pointing toward the toes. Keep hands firm as they have to support your whole body. Now raise the knees, lower the abdomen and slowly begin to stretch your legs. The body is actually supported on the elbows (Figure 63–1).

c.   Hold for a few seconds and rest before you attempt to raise your body again.

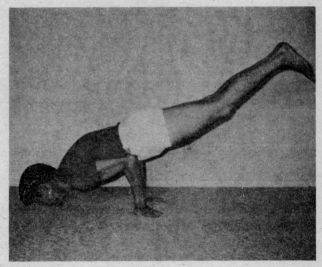

Figure 63–1

Crow Pose—Kakasana

a.   Sit on toes, knees apart, hands firmly on the floor.

b.   Inhale, and raise the toes, keeping them up for a while (Figure 64–1).

c.   Exhale and return to the starting position. Repeat a few times.

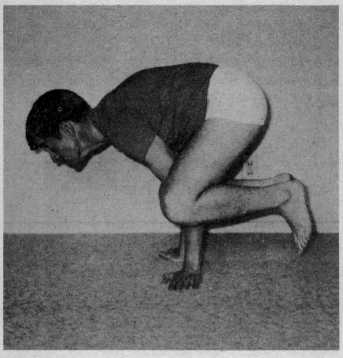

Figure 64–1

Leg Stretching Pose for Advanced Students

a.   Sit on the floor.

b.   Bend the right knee. Hold the thigh with your arm and then clasp the hands in the back (Figure 65–1). Sit briefly in this position and do the deep breathing. Alternate and then relax.

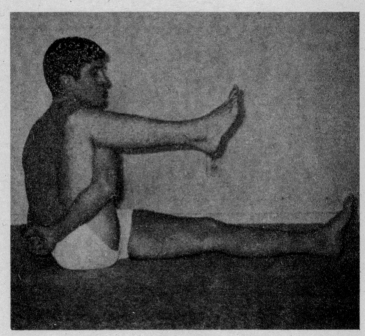

Figure 65–1

Advanced Shoulderstand Pose

Shoulderstand demonstrated by Tom Abbott. Description of this exercise can be found on page 122.

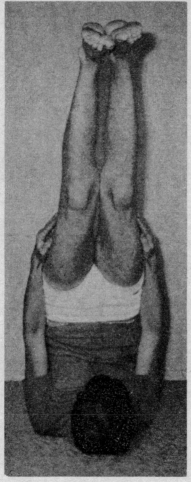

Figure 66–1

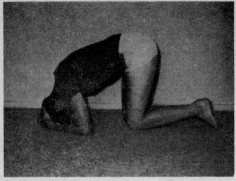

Figure 67-1

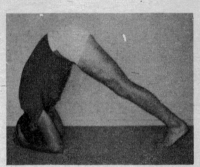

Figure 67-2

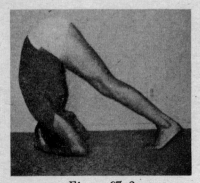

Figure 67-3

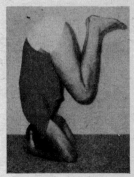

Figure 67-4

Another demonstration of a headstand as done by Tom Abbott

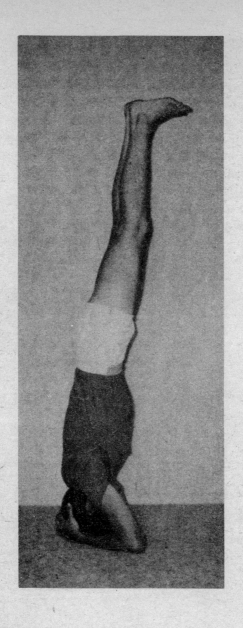

Lion Pose—Simhasan

a.   Sit in a kneeling position, palms over the knees, fingers apart and tensed.

b.   Stretch the tongue as far out as possible, eyes open wide. Lean forward and stiffen your body (Figure 68–1).

c.   Inhale, and then, pushing the tongue out, exhale making a peculiar sound of aaaaaaaaaa. Repeat this exercise three to six times.

This posture relieves the tension in the throat. Students who occasionally get sore throats, feel much better after this exercise. The tongue must be stretched out, in order to promote the circulation to the root of the throat.

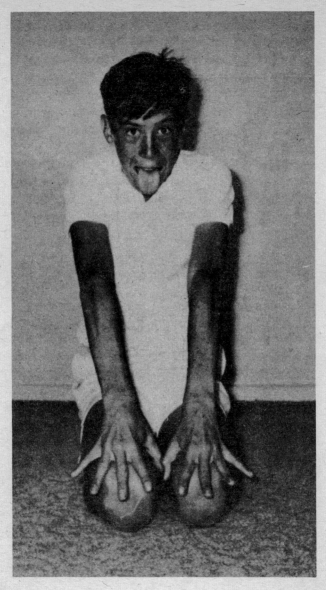

Figure 68–1   Chris Dunn

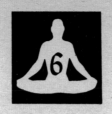

Guide to Mental and
Physical Health

OUR BODIES

Our glands, muscles, nerves, cells and blood circulation all have jobs to perform. When you understand their functions, you will not abuse your body, nor undermine the necessity of taking good care of it.

There are a number of glands in the human body and they are all interrelated: the *pituitary gland* is greatly responsible for body growth; the *pineal gland* controls the harmony of the other glands; the *thyroid gland* controls our inner activity and is responsible for our moods and mental alertness; the *parathyroid glands* when they function properly bring a balance to the body and provide it with a sense of peace; the *thymus gland* is actually active only during our childhood and is rather insignificant when one reaches puberty; the *adrenal gland* is responsible for our inner energy and many of our activities; the *gonads, or sex glands* when they work properly show in our personality, and even go as far as to express self-assurance and outer beauty.

Thus we cannot speak of the role of any particular gland, as they don't function separately. There is a definite well-ordered system of glands and their main duty is to control, to coordinate, to preserve unity and harmony in the human body.

The vitality of man depends on the condition of his endocrine glands at a given moment. Weakness of these glands bring, as a rule, a decrease of vitality, a breakdown of the human organism. The glands produce internal secretions known as hormones which are passed into the bloodstream, and in this way permeate all parts of the body. The bloodstream is a two-way lifeline, circulating throughout the body. During its course it affects the functioning of every organ, tissue, cell, bone, gland and nerve in the entire system. The stream flows through veins, arteries and

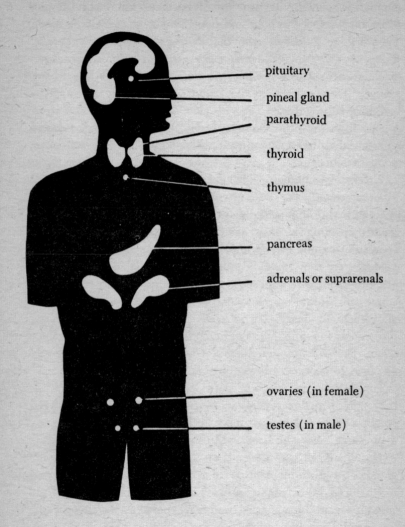

pituitary

pineal gland

parathyroid

thyroid

thymus

pancreas

adrenals or suprarenals

ovaries (in female)

testes (in male)

capillaries, making its way to all parts of the body. In one direction it carries oxygen and nourishment to every cell; along the other line it carries away the waste products sloughed off by living tissues. The bloodstream is a protective force, composed of countless sentinels striving to maintain a normally functioning system. The condition of the blood can spell the clue to your well-being.

The deep rhythmic breathing practiced with the yoga postures brings additional oxygen into the blood, helping its purification, and in turn removes all obstacles interfering with a proper blood supply to the glands, which in turn re-establishes their normal activity. Therefore it is essential to do your yoga exercises daily and learn the deep breathing properly. But, we also have to remember that the body needs nourishing foods, so that the glands are well nourished to produce the secretions, or hormones.

SUGGESTIONS FOR COMFORTABLE, RESTFUL AND HEALTHFUL SLEEP

1. The bed should be arranged so that the head is toward the north. The window should be left open to get plenty of fresh air into the lungs during the rest period. However, if the weather is damp, foggy, or cold, the window should be only slightly open. Avoid keeping flowers or any kind of green plants in the room at night.
2. Avoid soft mattresses or too many pillows. Keep the room dark, and if there is light coming in from the outside, cover the eyes with a light-weight dark scarf.
3. Try to get about seven hours of restful sleep. Apparently our bodies don't require more than that amount to receive sufficient rest. In fact, an article in *Newsweek*, of October

28th, 1968, reveals very exciting facts. It stated: "At a symposium at Albany Medical College, Dr. E. Guyler Hammond of the ACS reported that heart attacks and stroke deaths increase with the number of hours a person sleeps." Study which began in 1958 and various experiments on a large number of people led Dr. Hammond to this idea and he thinks that prolonged sleeping could be a symptom of arterosclerosis: ". . . that is, as the arteries narrow and the circulation of the brain becomes sluggish, the level of consciousness would be affected. In the latter case, long sleep sessions could cause heart attacks and strokes by slowing down the circulation and increaing the risk of clots in the heart or brain."

The Yogis claim that the body doesn't require too much sleep, as long as it has a quiet and peaceful rest. A few hours should be enough to refresh the body with new energy and strength. Thus they had this idea thousands of years ago. Recently, we are beginning to appreciate the old fashioned Yogic principles and philosophy and are adding them to our daily life.

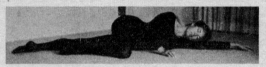

Sleeping Position—Dradhasana

a.   Lie down on your right side.
b.   The left leg is stretched and the right one bent over, arms stretched comfortably (as pictured).

This is the way the Yogis suggested we should sleep at night for better circulation. It is a very relaxing pose. At start, it might not feel comfortable, but once mastered this position brings a restful sleep, with no weight on the heart. I, personally, am so comfortable in this position, I can't sleep any other way.

Physical exercises and *Mental* exercises are interwoven so closely that *one* cannot function well without the *other*. You cannot succeed in gaining mental control without muscular relaxation. The body and mind are one! It is easier to relieve tension through relaxation of the muscles than to try to do it mentally.

Doctors tell us that many diseases arise from mental non-balance caused by stress, fear and confusion of the mind. The muscles and nerves are tense when you get angry or upset. Indeed, the anxieties of the "inner" man brought about by exaggerated mental and emotional pressures of the "outer" man often explode into complete mental or physical collapse. Our modern society brings these intense pressures to bear on man virtually every day of his adult life! Where can he turn for escape?

The Yoga technique of relaxation deserves serious consideration. Systematic relaxation of the muscles and mind through Hatha-Yoga relaxation exercises once or twice a day, on awakening and retiring, will pay dividends of well-being and peace. These methods, inspired by natural habits, are fundamentally based on concentration and relaxation; rhythm of breath and rhythm of the body. The *relaxation method* assures that the body grows stronger and the mind calmer as man acquires the know-how to remain happy and healthy in the feverish excitement of his busy life.

The spiritual element is lacking in the life of modern man, without which the other elements cannot be brought into harmony, for it is only in seeing man as a spiritual creature that we recognize how harmonious he may be.

The practice of relaxing every muscle brings rest to the body and mind. Eventually the tension will be relieved and you will not waste any energy. Those who know how to relax can close their eyes for a few minutes and do the mental relaxation any time; without any preparation, simply "let go." During that short period the entire system is re-charged, like a new battery, energy and vigor flowing into every organ, muscle and nerve.

UPON RISING

Upon arising, don't jump out of bed rapidly. Take time to stretch, bringing the body gradually to life again. Still in bed, flat on your back, do the complete stretching exercise. Start with one leg stretching slowly out, counting "One-two-three-four-five," up to ten, to begin with. Then bring the leg back and do the same with the other leg. Add one count every day until you count to thirty. Stretching builds control of muscles.

Then slowly get out of bed, first putting down one leg, then the other. Stand straight, arms above the head, and stretch the whole body (Figure a). Next start swinging to the right and then to the left (Figure b). Repeat a few times.

Then bring your hands down and start swinging the body from left to right, lifting the heel of the opposite foot, keeping the toe on the floor (Figure c). The head, eyes, and arms should follow the motion of the body with perfect ease and without any strain. The body and mind should relax with the rhythm of the swinging.

MENTAL AND PHYSICAL RELAXATION

A great deal of physical strain is imposed on us by the life we lead. Man through modern living has forgotten nature's rules on how to breathe correctly; indeed, he is not even aware of the necessity of breathing correctly. He has brought tension to his body through wrong habits, but he has not learned how to undo it.

Rhythmic breathing and relaxation enable you to overcome muscular tension and mental strain and fatigue. Yoga helps to restore the normal working order of the entire organism, and relaxation of body and mind go hand in hand with health, youth, happiness and long life. It is amazing what a few minutes of quiet can do for the body when left motionless, giving the muscles and nerves a chance to rest.

The Hunza people, known to have such unusual endurance, practice the science of relaxation, whether they know it or not. One can see them sitting absolutely motionless during meditation or prayers, without tension on their faces. Everything they do is done without tension, in a very relaxed manner. They don't hurry, but work is well organized and they don't lose any time, and *never* get panicky. You can observe that perfect *calmness within*.

Method of Physical Relaxation

1. The best position is to lie down on your back on the floor. If this is difficult for you, a couch or bed will do.
2. Bear in mind that you must relax every part of the body, beginning with the toes and ending with the head.
3. Keep both hands loose at your sides.
4. Close your eyes.
5. Now begin to relax the toes, then the ankles, knees, thighs, hips, and spinal cord.
6. Relax your shoulders, arms, forearms, elbows, wrists, hands, and fingers.
7. Now relax your head, your facial muscles; drop your chin.
8. You are now completely relaxed.
9. Keep in mind the picture of calmness. You are completely relaxed, completely at peace.

Method of Mental Relaxation

1. After every muscle in your body is relaxed and the mind calm, think of something pleasant. Remember that you must keep your mind free from any disturbing thoughts in order for it to relax.
2. Create a beautiful scene in your mind: think of the majestic Himalayan Mountains, of a magnificent sunset or a blue sky with milky clouds. Imagine yourself floating on one of these clouds over vast lakes, fields, gardens. See only pictures of beauty and feel that life is pulsating through you. Remain in this position for five to ten minutes.
3. Start stretching, first the arms, then the legs.
4. Roll to one side, then to the other.
5. Yawn a few times and open eyes.
6. Slowly sit up, not to break the spell of the benefits you have derived.

This method should follow your daily physical exercises. But it also can be done during the day. It is advisable for a business man, for instance, to take a few minutes from work, lock the door of his office, and relax. The mind will rest from the strain, overworked muscles will quiet down. These few minutes will rejuvenate the whole being, giving you peace of mind.

The secretary, the saleslady, the factory worker—anyone, without exception—can find a quiet corner during the luncheon hour, and if you cannot stretch out on the floor, sit in a chair or on a bench in a park to do the exercises.

Very few women have learned the art of resting; consequently, many of them constantly complain of being tired. This tiredness is caused by nervous tension, which directly affects their beauty. To avoid this a woman should devote some time each day to relaxation exercises.

Vocal Exercises

The Yogis have devised special sounds called "mantras," which are based on certain vowel combinations. The mantras are chanted in a certain manner so as to produce a vibrating effect on the entire system: the nerves, glands, and brain. The Hunza people chant every morning and evening during their prayers. They practice these mantras, absolutely unaware of the effects they have on their health.

The mantras are done in the following manner:

1. Inhale first; then, without exhaling, sound a strong and piercing "EEEEEEEEEEEEEEEEEE," holding the mouth as in a smile. The sound should be even and kept on the same pitch. Stop before you are out of breath. Inhale again and repeat the same vowel. The vibration will be in your ears.

2. Follow the same routine with other vowels, such as "AAAAAAAAAAAAAAAA," which will vibrate in your throat.

3. "OOOOOOOOOOOOOOOOOOOOO"—with this sound you will feel the vibration in your chest.

4. "UUUUUUUUUUUUUUUUUUUU"—with this sound you will feel the vibration in your stomach.

5. Use the vowels together: "OOOUUUOOOUUU"; "AAA-AAAAAAAAAAOOOOOOOOOOOO"; "MMMMMMMMOOO-OOO"; "MOMOMOMOMOMOMOMOMOMOMO"; OMOM-OMOMOMOM."

Ideally, these vocal exercises should follow the relaxation exercises just described. They can also be done at any time during the day when you have a free moment.

CONCENTRATION AND MEDITATION EXERCISES

Yoga is the philosophy which teaches the unity of life or the oneness of consciousness. It elevates the mind to magnificent heights of divine splendor and glory, which makes man absolutely fearless, which destroys all barriers that separate man from man and which brings peace and harmony to suffering humanity.

Yoga is the philosophy of life which if practiced by the majority could bring harmony among families, and harmony between nations. Yoga builds an inner spiritual strength, develops infinite knowledge and inspires, invigorates and puts a stop to negativeness.

I once heard a great man say: "If we unite nations we can hope for eternal peace." But how can it be accomplished unless the individual has found unity within himself?

Concentration is fixing the mind on a point or an object, either internal or external. Meditation is surrounding that one thing or idea with the flow of continuous thought.

Meditation and concentration exercises have a powerful influence on the mind, nerves, organs and cells of the body. Yogis who meditate regularly are known to have strong, healthy bodies and Divine nature. The ability to concentrate and meditate is a wonderful experience, but it requires training. I remember hearing a lecturer speaking on meditation say, "We *think* that we think, but only a handful of people really know how to concentrate on one thought at one time and keep the thought on that particular object or subject."

The mind is a mischievous imp, it is jumpy, and must be disciplined daily to bring it under control. Therefore it is urgent that you begin to practice daily concentration and meditation to learn to control your mind. The mind is a combination of feeling, knowledge and willingness. You can use either of these aspects in such a manner that the mind can be directed to that particular point which you have chosen.

Concentration to keep the mind on one point at a time is the beginning of the exercise.

1. Choose the time for meditation when your mind is clear and calm. Then find a quiet place, some corner where you are not going to be disturbed for a while.

2. Sit at ease and close your eyes. (The Yogis use the Lotus pose for meditation as they claim that in this position you can be completely relaxed and keep your spine straight.)

3. Forget everything around you. Silence the thoughts. Forget the body.

4. Breathe slowly. Feel joy and bliss.

5. Fill the mind with beautiful thoughts and allow no other thought or idea to enter your mind or disturb you.

6. Put your mind on one thing and keep it on this one subject or object, no matter what it is. If you picture a flower, stick to the flower; don't suddenly jump to another object. Try to see all the beautiful flowers in your mind until they are as clear as though you are actually seeing a garden with flowers.

7. Allow no other thought or idea to disturb it. Concentrate on the thought you have chosen and direct all its power into that one channel. As soon as you are able to concentrate you have gained the power of doing things. Through the power of concentration and meditation it is possible to develop a will to function in a world of peace and happiness combined with a healthy body.

8. Concentration is a powerful weapon, but be aware which direction your thoughts have taken.

9. In meditation you really don't ask for anything. Swami Sivananda calls meditation "the flow of continuous thought or one thing or God."

10. You can concentrate and meditate with results only after your physical body has been brought to perfection.
11. After you have accomplished the requirements, you can start meditating on various ideas, but be careful in choosing your wishes and desires. Always keep in mind to ask yourself, "Is this right for me?" Remember that whatever you ask will come into your life—so don't ask for anything you couldn't cope with!

Swami Paramananda, in *Concentration and Meditation,* writes: "One who has not proper control over his body cannot make proper use of his mind. He can never concentrate—much less can he meditate. A man who lacks mastery over his physical organism cannot possibly gain spiritual consciousness."

WALKING EXERCISES AND THEIR BENEFITS

The medical profession has stressed the value of walking to maintain good health. Systematic exercising and walking bring the flow of oxygen into your blood to keep your system working and your body youthful.

1. Walk for about two or three miles daily. and even more if you don't feel fatigued.
2. Choose a proper rhythm or pace and maintain it during your entire walk. Tiredness can be caused by change of pace or rhythm.
3. Do the deep breathing exercises as you put the right foot in front of the left foot. Count one-two-three-four, in—and, one-two-three-four, out.
4. Do not continue to do the deep breathing exercises all the time. They should be done only a few times during the walk. The additional intake of oxygen might stimulate the brain too much and cause dizziness.

5. The duration of each step should harmonize with its length. Regulate the rhythm of your steps accordingly. This will be your natural walking rhythm which you should adopt and retain always, no matter how fast you walk.
6. Balance and rhythm in everything you do plays the predominant role in your life. The habit of doing it, after practicing for a while, will become an automatic matter, and save a lot of energy.

The Hunza people are the proof that walking is an excellent exercise. They walk up and down their hills without any effort and some of them walk for miles every day in one stretch without feeling fatigued.

SEX IS ART

The many divorces and marital problems are the proof that our world is in a confused state of mind. Observing the happy married couples in Hunza, I am prompted to discuss sex.

A Hunza woman is sure of her husband's love, and, in turn, she trusts him implicitly. A man has complete freedom of action and this freedom keeps him attached to his home, to his wife, and to his children, as he is made to believe that he is the leader.

But the woman is still the "queen" at home, not domineering, but kind and loving, and thus she has created a place for herself. The absence of jealousy and mistrust in a marriage makes it a beautiful institution. Doubt, stress, and jealousy have deprived many people of happiness.

The physical incapacity of a marital partner often leads to the separation of many couples. Man is born to possess the qualities of a monogamist and unless a woman finds a way to satisfy a man physically and hold him through physical and spiritual attraction, he will look for another mate.

Some women just love to criticize their husbands or sweethearts in front of others. A man cannot stand criticism; it hurts his ego. Build his ego in front of others, for a man loves to be flattered.

There is something else: the women of Hunza are very feminine. They don't neglect their appearance after getting married. They have lovely and healthy complexions which add to their beauty.

A woman who wants to keep her husband must be responsive, must be attractive, warm, and she has to accept the emotional atmosphere of her man. She has to learn to laugh when he laughs, and to enjoy life when he does. If she cares and wants to keep her man, she must always be right there when he needs her. She must be tender, feminine, intelligent, and build an inner security which protects her from being jealous and ugly.

It has been said that behind every successful man is a good woman. It is true, but only a clever woman can lead a man to success and draw out his best qualities.

A man will remain faithful to a woman he needs, because he will find the security he has been looking for. But today's newlyweds seem to give very little thought to actual marital life and the responsibilities connected with it.

Magazines, newspapers and television shows talk about the problems that sex is causing all over the world. While we hear constant protest, nothing tangible seems to have been accomplished to remedy this. Is it possible that most of the trouble has been caused by a misunderstanding of sex?

Sex education is given in school. Children are taught that sex is an internal part of marriage, that babies are conceived through the sexual union of man and woman and not brought by the stork. They are taught about their sex organs, about venereal disease and even study the development of a human embryo. Fifteen-year-old girls of today know that when they have intercourse with their boy friends there is a great chance of pregnancy. Yet the rate of illegitimate births is an established fact. The problems are not inadequate sex education, but our attitude toward sex. We no longer think of "sex and marriage" as one. We think of sex and then if love comes along, marriage, too. Sex is love to some of us. However, they forgot one thing; that sex is no game. The sexual compatibility of a man and woman cannot be achieved on "one night stands."

A woman must protect her integrity and self-respect if she wants to be respected by a man. A doctor told me some drastic facts about young girls who become pregnant. These girls are so ignorant that it is pathetic, he told me. They are not aware in the least what it is all about. The youngest are fourteen. A moment of physical satisfaction, the girl gets pregnant and the boy has disappeared out of her life.

Isn't it up to the parents to control such emotions? Setting the example at home of respectable behavior should be the first thing in the upbringing of the child. As a rule in a happy and contented home, out-of-wedlock pregnancy doesn't happen as often as among couples who haven't found contentment and happiness themselves.

Another important factor is that when sex is regarded as something to be ashamed of, inhibitions set into the mind of a young person. When such a woman gets married, she knows little about sexual satisfaction during her close relationship with her husband. After a while, she doesn't understand why she is irritable, worried, unhappy and fearful of losing her husband. Because of the inability to establish a sexually harmonious union, soon he, too, becomes restless.

Doctor Benjamin Spock, writes in an article, "How Parents Can Help Adolescents Understand Sex," in *Reader's Digest*, September, 1962, "One particularly confusing aspect of sex is that, at different times, many adults take differing attitudes toward it. At one time they will talk as if it were almost sacred, then as if it were shameful, then again as if it were a joke to snicker at. This gives a teen-ager the impression that adults are hypocrites and makes his own understanding of sex more difficult. It seems to be hard for us to think of sex as both natural and noble. Some teen-agers conclude that sex and love are just a matter of biology."

Of course, there are instances when the man thinks of sex as his act of pleasure, and worries little about satisfying his wife. The first steps of sexual maturity are terribly important. They build the basic pattern of future life, and many divorces could be avoided if our young people would be taught the facts of life in its true sense of the word. Knowledge is truth—and truth means freedom from fear! There is no reason why any child, no matter how young, should not receive honest answers to his questions about sex.

My definition of sex is, "Sex is art," and if it would be treated as *art*, the world might face less problems concerning sexual stability.

Some men worry that as they grow older they will become unable to satisfy a woman sexually. A man may become so haunted by lack of self-assurance that he becomes impotent. It is not years that make us old—years alone do not lessen the ability of sexual powers—it is what the individual does to his body, by acquiring bad habits, wrong foods, wrong thinking, lack of exercise.

The Hunzas have shown us that age has nothing to do with physical manifestations. The man of eighty years old can experience the emotions of a twenty-year-old. It is our thinking that begins the decline. Thus reach within you and there you will find the rich qualities of health, love, peace and faith.

OLD AGE

Today the average person between forty and fifty dreads the approach of old age. Without exception, we are trying to conceal gray hair, wrinkles and sagging lines, and extra pounds, but the look of anxiety on the face cannot be concealed. The fear of old age creeps in, bringing unhappiness and a negative outlook on life.

"How old are you?" seems to be such an important question. No person with imagination need ever grow old; the secret of youthfulness is in our own keeping. Life is a matter of going forward. A mind kept vital by a spirit of enthusiasm and desire for new adventure has found the secret of eternal youth. Youth is an expression of life, and life is eternal.

Life is only beginning at forty or fifty. There is so much to learn it requires time to get ready for it. Scientists are beginning to be aware that life is an endless process of growth, and our cells are continually being renewed. Why, then, should cells be replaced by old or deficient ones? Life is a perpetual process of tearing down and building up. It has perfect balance, but human ignorance and error have interfered with its rhythmic equilibrium.

The Yogis believe that there is no natural death and man dies because he lost the secret of eternal life. They also believe that anyone who can master the higher teachings of Yoga can live indefinitely; however, they do eventually die, for the reason that they believe their job on earth has been accomplished and they are ready for a rest—rather a higher stage of evolution.

Man has to acquire the know-how to live a longer life, but unless he enjoys good health, there is no reason for him to live. The moment man cannot be useful and active, he merely exists and vegetates instead of living. People can be fit and active at almost any age, as has been proven by a few exceptional men and women who are living to 100 and older in perfect mental condition.

The subject of youth has intrigued me ever since I was a young girl. I couldn't accept the theory that I have to grow old because the calendar keeps moving ahead. Because of the sun making an evolution around the earth, I am supposed to add one day to my body, and then 365 days will make me one year older. To me it was sheer nonsense. I was aware that I couldn't always be young looking, but at least I can keep fit and active as long as I am alive.

Since I became interested in yoga and began to practice its technique, and then was fortunate enough to learn the great truth about the Hunza people, which led me to change my old habits and follow their diet, way of living and thinking, I have not felt a single day older. In fact, I feel better now than when I began my program.

Today I am awake, alert and alive, and am able to exercise and participate in many sports such as bowling, swimming, walking. My mind is at peace and I have learned the spiritual value of life, and I have been able to recognize what peace of mind means in its truest sense. Before I stumbled on the combined philosophy of Hunza-Yoga, unhappy thoughts were deeply planted into my soul, leaving me no choice but to feel miserable. But then I became aware that my consciousness was asleep!

I am afraid that until nations wake up to the truth and dare to admit that the deterioration of the physical, mental and spiritual aspects of man are the result of our state of mind we'll continue to look for solutions to the sorry state of the world. Man is blind and doesn't want to recognize that the answers are within himself!

Yogis say that old age is a state of mind. When you begin to feel old, you are old. Many men and women did their best work at fifty and later. Goethe wrote the second part of Faust at eighty-two. If you feel old at sixty, then you have indulged in the wrong habits and abused your body. You are as old as you feel, as old as your thoughts, and as old as your doubts.

Don't get discouraged when your children tell you that you are too old to play games, or wear certain clothes, or go dancing with them. Laugh it off—and prove to them that you can do all these things at all ages as well as they do. At the end they will have to accept you, because if you can prove your stamina and alertness, they will be proud of you!

The rules which the Yogis set up are simple:

1. Breathe plenty of fresh and pure air.
2. Eat natural foods and much of it in a raw stage. Don't overcook your food, otherwise the valuable ingredients of nutrients so essential to build a strong body will be destroyed.
3. Continue physical activities to keep the blood circulating, by walking, exercising, playing games, no matter how old you are.

Keep an interest in the world around you. Then bear in mind that happiness is another valuable factor in keeping young.

SMOKING AND YOGA

The report on "Smoking and Health," made to the Surgeon General of the United States by an expert advisory committee, said that many people with emphysema are heavy smokers, and that there is a relationship between cigarette smoking and the disease. The Surgeon General's report says, "The smoking of cigarettes is associated with an increased risk of dying from pulmonary (lung) emphysema." It is definite, experts believe, that cigarette smoking is a major cause of the distressing symptoms of chronic bronchitis.

How smoking harms the lungs is far from clear. But one thing is known: cigarette smoke interferes with the lungs' cleaning system. This system works by means of hairlike projections that line the air tubes. They rid the lungs of outside matter brought in with the air by keeping up a steady movement upward—that is, from the insides of the lungs outward. In this way the layer of mucous that the bronchial lining secretes is kept moving upward and outward, into the windpipe and throat, where it is either spit out or swallowed harmlessly. A great deal of the matter gets into the lungs with air—dust, germs and the like—is caught in the mucous and carried out of the air tubes of the lungs along with it.

Interference with this natural cleaning process obviously has its dangers. The particles of dirt from polluted air, as well as germs, get a chance to do damage if they are not removed promptly and efficiently. Thus, its slowing-down effect on the moving, hairlike "brooms" of the air tubes is one way that cigarette smoking can very probably be harmful to the lungs.

In addition, dryness in the tubes and tissues is a part of the trouble for many patients with breathing problems. Smoking tends to increase such dryness.

"Another thing proves the bad effects of cigarette smoking," a doctor told his patient. "If you will stop smoking tomorrow, I can almost guarantee that you will have less trouble with your breathing within a few days or weeks." When a patient is found to have a chronic breathing disorder, especially emphysema, the first thing to be done is to stop his smoking, if he smokes—and almost invariably he feels better as a result.

PEACE OF MIND

The word "anxiety" has become a very popular word. Spiritual uncertainties have increased anxieties and fears and to conquer these complexities so that we may manage our lives with more wisdom and confidence we must learn to have more faith in God.

Many feel defeated when they are confronted with difficult tests, and stew over every problem. There is a way out of every situation, though our failures may be varied and numerous. Whatever we do represents the level of our understanding and development. A faulty judgment is made only because of too little experience, but you should never lose faith in your ability. Lack of understanding of a certain matter doesn't prove ignorance.

Within all of us is a well-meaning spirit. We are all striving toward the goal of perfection, but when you fail don't ever say that you have no faith. Faith is a wonderful thing. It is the very substance of things desired. But faith must be grounded in love and hope.

Faith stirs the mind to hold to the belief that all things are possible. Hope quickens expectancy and clears the vision. All negative emotions and states of mind must be swept out, and the tools with which this can be accomplished are faith, love, understanding, forgiveness, and they will bring us to the environment of complete peace of mind. Right thinking and constructive action will clear out the residue of discontent and all the other dark thoughts that choke the inflow of vigor and health into the body, and will contribute to our finding that illusive thing called peace.

When love rules your life and mind, greed, envy, fear, hate or possessiveness have no place for destructive growth.

Consciousness is a directing power in the mind itself. Thought is governed by law, and lack of understanding causes people to lose faith in the Divine Law.

Fear of situation will bring fear. And if you dwell on a subject which has been created by your personal confusion and fear it will increase your confusion and soon you will begin to believe in the danger around you.

To train your thinking, start believing that your mind works with the precision of the law of electricity. There is no explanation to it, but it functions. You know you have to turn the switch on to get light, and flick it off when you don't need light any longer. The same happens to your mind. You can feed it with love or fear. When you understand this you will accept that good health, happiness and prosperity are conditioned to your own thinking. Consciously or unconsciously you must accept the theory that thoughts are born in the mind, and their offspring express what you originally planted—in other words, practice mental exercises to train the mind to accept only loving, harmonious and beautiful thoughts. Mental exercises are just as essential as physical exercises. Relaxation techniques can help rid you of emotions which at the end only destroy your well-being.

Dr. Frank N. Allan, a Boston internist, in a study determined that almost 80 per cent of his patients were tired or feeling restless because of emotional difficulties. "A study of chronically tired business executives in their early forties and fifties was made at a Chicago hospital. These men had been full of driving ambition, eager to accept responsibilities, determined to reach the top. But somewhere along the way they had lost their drive, their incentive to work. All were thoroughly discouraged and terribly tired. 'It seemed that their mainsprings were broken,' observed one physician."

Extreme exhaustion is caused by lack of a positive attitude. When you do something because you believe in it, because you want to do it, you can foresee the successful outcome of it without fear creeping into your subconscious mind. Doubt and insecurity sap your energy and make you tired. Worry and fear are ravenous creatures who have made their way into our society and modern living and have become irritants to the mind and body.

God created man in His own image and invested him with many qualities and abilities, among them the spiritual power to fulfill his purpose on earth. He has given us all we need to achieve a happy life, establish peace, health, harmony, abundance and order. Worry, however, has succeeded in infiltrating every nation save one, the land of Hunza.

A wonderful feeling of peace prevails in Hunza: a feeling of direct contact with God. Peace, harmony and the spirit of love are enjoyed there. These people are free from regrets of the past and apprehension about the future. They carry out their daily chores quietly, without stress or strain, without nervous tension. Therefore, when the job is completed, it is done well and efficiently. There is a purpose in their every movement and in their every job.

The people of Hunza can show us the way to Peace of Mind if we let them. Nowhere in the world are there happier people. They have built a pattern of thought which has created a satisfying, purposeful life. Indeed, the Hunzakuts have found happiness and prosperity—prosperity in the true riches of life: love, peace of mind, health, and spiritual understanding.

POSITIVE THINKING

Our thoughts are instrumental in everything we try to do. Thus if you are depressed today because something unpleasant has happened to you, begin to work on your thoughts in the opposite direction and your problem will take on a different shape.

Consider yourself the mechanism of your body. Feeling is a mental reaction and precedes the definite thought. If you permit your feeling to be depressed for a period of time, eventually it will trap you into negative channels. True, you have not consciously invited trouble, but there is a chance you formed it with your own imagination that something is wrong or will go wrong. And what your mind imagines, sooner or later comes into expression.

You are governed by your feelings much more than you are aware. You and I are swayed by likes and dislikes. For instance, perhaps sometime in your life you had a grudge against someone you knew; later you learned that his affairs went wrong, and this gave you a feeling of joy, of satisfaction that he met his punishment. Be careful what you think concerning others as the same might take shape in your own life, because you are releasing a negative thought pattern ready to be brought forth into expression. Don't entertain a thought that you would not like to happen in your own life. Remember you are merely what your thoughts assemble.

The scientist tells us that we live in the Universal ether. It is formless, but it forms around us according to our thoughts. Our conscious mind is the central point from which thoughts flow and therefore we have to become aware of our consciousness and of our thoughts and realize that we are creating causes which have an effect on our environment and our bodies. These effects are set into action by our own thinking and expressions. The scientific world has become aware that behind everything is the wonderful instrument of the *mind*.

Thoughts flow into the ether all day long and they are picked up by others as ideas which come to mind from nowhere. Therefore, you have to be very careful in letting destructive thoughts into the ether, because these thoughts have a magnetic power to return to you. "Like attracts like!" The mind can cope only with one situation at a time; as you consciously supply it with beauty and love, destructive habits which have been influencing your actions are eliminated. Right now is a good time to begin! Instead of letting your moods possess and rule you, take command of them!

We must be diligent, watchful of our emotions and our thoughts. As we exercise our bodies to keep physically fit, so must our mental and emotional nature be constantly kept in good condition. The cleansing and dynamic power of right ideas and of high and ennobling thoughts is of inestimable value, not only in keeping our own spiritual channel open, but in helping others to find truth and peace of mind.

How marvelous it would be if destructive ideas and negative words never entered our thinking! But they do, and when they do we must eliminate them. We must keep working at it and keep our spiritual consciousness clear of resentment, worry, anger, selfishness and fear.

Words are the outer expression of *thought*, so it is obvious that we must give a great deal of attention to the disciplining of our thoughts. By the power of thought we not only form states of mind in ourselves, but we also surround ourselves with a thought atmosphere which, in turn, affects the order of the world. We must create thoughts of peace and beauty to send into the atmosphere if we want better world-wide conditions.

If you had a way of recording every thought that goes through your mind just for one day, it would prove to you the theory of the necessity to train your mind to accept positive thinking. It would demonstrate why one day is pleasant and another full of disappointments. Your emotions and thoughts are mixed—a combination of good and, at the same time, selfish and fearful thoughts. This explains why we say words we don't mean; why illness strikes suddenly; why disharmony pervades our lives instead of peace. All the conditions that we do not like have been brought about by our own thinking and they can be remedied only as we discipline our thoughts along true lines.

Don't let anybody tell you that your mind is not capable of change. Don't blame fate for the shift in your life, because only *you* control it. One of the greatest hindrances to progress is making excuses for shortcomings, instead of facing them. It is much more sensible to use the energy to correct the mistake than to make excuses for it.

If someone criticizes you, don't get angry. If the criticism was justified, although you didn't agree at the time and fought your conviction, try not to judge the person. Instead, examine the issue quietly to make sure who was right and who was wrong. But don't ever keep a grudge against truth. On the other hand, if you should be accused of something of which you are not guilty, try to understand the other person instead of resenting him. Understanding is the goal for which you should strive, and don't let criticism dampen your spirits or lessen your courage to carry out your convictions. Criticism might also be of great help; it might lead you to analyze carefully your motives and actions.

There is one thing to bear in mind: you live your *own* life. You are the mirror of your own thoughts, your own words, your own actions. Your life is a result of what you think—in fact, it *is* what you think! Therefore you must train your mind to think constructively, as thoughts produce their own images in the material world.

True, thought habits are like any other habits, requiring training, but you can learn to control them and guide them. If undesirable thoughts invade your mind, get busy putting it in order without delay. You are in command of your life and only *you* have command of your thoughts. Face life with courage and confidence. The world is yours, awaiting your recognition and your use.

You can use this form of training. Write these things out, read them daily and put them into practice:

1. Choose what you desire.
2. Cleanse yourself of everything that would be in your way.
3. Claim it to be yours already.
4. Believe that it is yours now in spirit.
5. Give thanks for it.
6. It will come to pass.

You can also draw pictures of the things you would like to have or possess. But never ask for anything beyond your capacity to handle. Ask in moderation, with humility.

Some people have made scrap books of pictures from magazines of the things that they desire. Look at them, think and work toward getting what you have asked for.